LIMITED
RADIOGRAPHY

Second Edition

DEDICATION

To my mother, who was my best friend and whose loving care and sustained support always gave me the courage and the drive to meet my goals.

Frances E. Campeau

To my family and loved ones: Jennifer Phelps, Don Moore, Deanna and Charlie Hansen, and my parents, Jeanette and Joseph Fleitz and especially my grandparents who gave me a special kind of love, Kathleen and Joe Fleitz.

Jeana Fleitz

LIMITED RADIOGRAPHY

Second Edition

Frances E. Campeau

Jeana Fleitz

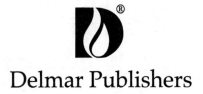

Delmar Publishers

an International Thomson Publishing company I(T)P®

Albany • Bonn • Boston • Cincinnati • Detroit • London • Madrid
Melbourne • Mexico City • New York • Pacific Grove • Paris • San Francisco
Singapore • Tokyo • Toronto • Washington

NOTICE TO THE READER

Cover Design: Charles Cummings Advertising/Art, Inc.

Delmar Staff:

Publisher: Susan Simpfenderfer
Acquisitions Editor: Marlene McHugh Pratt
Developmental Editor: Melissa Riveglia
Production Coordinator: William Trudell

Art and Design Coordinator: Rich Killar
Marketing Manager: Darryl L. Caron
Editorial Assistant: Maria Perretta

COPYRIGHT © 1998
By Delmar Publishers
an International Thomson Publishing company I(T)P®

The ITP logo is a trademark under license
Printed in the United States of America

For more information, contact:

Delmar Publishers
3 Columbia Circle, Box 15015
Albany, New York 12212-5015

International Thomson Publishing Europe
Berkshire House 168-173
168-173 High Holborn
London, WC1V 7AA
United Kingdom

Nelson ITP, Australia
102 Dodds Street
South Melbourne,
Victoria, 3205 Australia

Nelson Canada
1120 Birchmont Road
Scarborough, Ontario
M1K 5G4, Canada

International Thomson Publishing France
Tour Maine-Montparnasse
33 Avenue du Maine
75755 Paris Cedex 15, France

International Thomson Editores
Seneca 53
Colonia Polanco
11560 Mexico D. F. Mexico

International Thomson Publishing GmbH
Königswinterer Straße 418
53227 Bonn
Germany

International Thomson Publishing Asia
60 Albert Street
#15-01 Albert Complex
Singapore 189969

International Thomson Publishing Japan
Hirakawa-cho Kyowa Building, 3F
2-2-1 Hirakawa-cho, Chiyoda-ku,
Tokyo 102, Japan

ITE Spain/Parninfo
Calle Magallanes, 25
28015-Madrid, España

All rights reserved. No part of this work covered by the copyright hereon may be reproduced or used in any form or by any means — graphic, electronic, or mechanical, including photocopying, recording, taping, or information storage and retrieval systems — without the written permission of the publisher.

1 2 3 4 5 6 7 8 9 10 XXX 03 02 01 99 98

Library of Congress Cataloging-in-Publication Data
Campeau, Frances.
    Limited radiography / Frances E. Campeau, M. Jeana Fleitz. — 2nd ed.
        p. cm.
    Includes bibliographical references and index.
    ISBN 0-7668-0205-1
    1. Radiography, Medical.   2. Radiologic technologists.   3. Allied
health personnel.   I. Fleitz, M. Jeana. II. Title.
4. Technology, Radiologic.   WN 100 C193L 1998]
RC78.C33   1998
616.07'572—dc21
DNLM/DLC
for Library of Congress   98-27596
                                                                                                          CIP

Contents

Contents

Index of Tables

Preface

The radiography professions have seen many changes since Congress passed the Consumer-Patient Radiation Health and Safety Act (Public Law 97-35). The Act requires the Secretary of Health and Human Services to develop minimum standards for state accreditation of radiologic technology education programs and state certification or licensure of persons who administer ionizing and/or non-ionizing radiation in medical and dental radiologic procedures.

For many years, the radiologic technologist was the only level of worker who was tested and credentialed. The radiologic technologist completed a two-year program approved by the Committee on Allied Health Education Accreditation (CAHEA). As a result of Public Law 97-35, many states have adopted education and certification standards for radiation workers other than the two-year radiographers. These other workers are often known as limited radiographers and their work status varies from state to state. They are usually employed in physicians' offices, chiropractic and dental clinics, and in ambulatory care settings.

In 1985, the American Registry of Radiologic Technologists (ARRT) identified a task listing and began development of an examination that can be used by states that license limited radiographers. The ARRT indicates that the depth of required knowledge is the same for both limited and general radiographers; it is the scope of practice that differentiates the levels of radiographers.

The goal of this text is to meet the needs of the radiographer in limited practice and to upgrade the performance standards in these areas of practice. The authors have designed the text for students at the post-secondary level who plan to test for certification in limited radiography. It is also an excellent reference for medical workers who are participating in independent self-study programs for limited radiography.

The goal of the text is to provide students with a fundamental imaging foundation so that they are competent clinical practitioners capable of producing diagnostic radiographs while subjecting the patient and health care personnel to minimum radiation exposure.

The first three chapters introduce the student to radiography as a career. Topics covered include educational requirements, continuing education, professionalism, professional relationships, concepts for effective communication, and law and ethics.

Chapter 4 is concerned with medical aspects and patient care. The principles of infection control and universal precautions are stressed for the safety of the patient and health care workers. Basic concepts of patient care, including safety considerations and moving and transporting are also discussed.

Chapter 5 presents the basic concepts of radiation physics, beginning with the theory of atomic structure and continuing through the principles of electricity and magnetism. These concepts are then applied in Chapters 6–9, which are concerned with the technical aspects of radiography: production of radiation, imaging equipment, film exposure and film processing. Chapter 10 covers the evaluation of radiographic film images.

Chapters 11 and 12 are concerned with the safety of ionizing radiation. Chapter 11 covers the effect of ionizing radiation on human cells and tissues while Chapter 12 discusses radiation protection procedures and radiation detection and monitoring.

In selected chapters reference is made to specific tasks for which students of limited radiography must demonstrate competence. These tasks are outlined in the appendix. For each task, the following information is given: procedural title, terminal performance objective, a listing of equipment and supplies, and a performance guide (numbered sequential steps from the beginning to the end of the task).

The text does not discuss radiographic anatomy and positioning since there are many excellent texts available that deal in detail with these areas. The authors believe that by not "reinventing the wheel" they have been able to focus on the didactic presentation of radiographic imaging and radiation protection.

An Instructor's Manual accompanies the text. The manual includes answers to the chapter reviews and competency checklists for the procedural tasks listed in the text appendix.

Frances E. Campeau, MA, RT(R)(M), FAERS
Jeana Fleitz, MEd, RT(R)(M)

Acknowledgments

The idea for a textbook devoted to limited radiography has been in the minds of the authors for many years, long before its need became apparent. Planning a book and actually writing are two separate functions and the reality of bringing this book to fruition would not have been possible without certain other people.

We are forever indebted to Ms. Nancy C. Roubieu, whose enduring patience was responsible for the production of the manuscript and who was an indispensable editor.

Our friends and colleagues also have been supportive with ideas and just listening when it was needed.

Frances E. Campeau, MA, RT(R)(M), FAERS
Jeana Fleitz, MEd, RT(R)(M)

* * * * * * * *

The Delmar staff wishes to thank the professionals who reviewed the manuscript in its several stages. Appreciation for their constructive recommendations is extended to:

Cindy Lou Calhoun, CMA-CPT
Career Training Academy
New Kensington, PA

Margaret Hunkele, AS, RT(R)(M)(MRI)
Bryman School
Phoenix, AZ

Kenneth George, BA, RT(R)
SUNY Health Science Center
Syracuse, NY

Thomas Sandridge, BS, RT(R)
Miami-Dade Community College
Miami, FL

* * * * * * * *

The following companies provided technical information, illustrations and/or photographs.

Eastman Kodak Company
GE Medical Systems
IVAC Corporation

Chapter 1

Introduction to Limited Radiography: The Occupation

Chapter Outline

Introduction
History, Purpose, and Functions
   Philosophy Statement
   Occupational Scope and Purpose
Education
Continuing Education and Professional Organizations
Occupational Progress and Professionalization
The Future

Objectives

Upon completion of the chapter, the student will meet the following objectives by verifying knowledge of the facts and principles presented through oral and written communication at a level deemed competent.

1. Identify the occupational role and function of the limited radiographer.
2. Describe the impact of the Consumer-Patient Radiation Health and Safety Act on the development of the limited radiography occupation.
3. Discuss the role of continuing education in the professional growth and development of a limited radiographer.
4. List several prospects for employment as a limited radiographer.

INTRODUCTION

Does the term **limited radiography** designate a new occupation emerging within the radiological sciences, or does it designate a skill level within the radiological sciences consisting of limited radiography tasks performed by a myriad of workers in medical offices, clinics, and ambulatory care centers?

Why are individuals who operate radiation-producing equipment coming under state and federal guidelines and regulations that address the establishment of minimum educational standards, competency testing, and continuing education? Who are limited radiographers, how are they educated, and where are they employed? Do limited radiographers and radiologic technologists share a common professional role but differ in their level of responsibility and scope of practice? These are just a few of the many questions being asked today about limited radiography and individuals called limited radiographers. This chapter will focus on the essential characteristics of limited radiography as an occupation.

HISTORY, PURPOSE, AND FUNCTIONS

In November 1895, Wilhelm Conrad Roentgen announced his discovery of a new kind of radiant energy. Investigating conduction of electrons through a partially evacuated glass tube, he found that a plate coated with a fluorescent material emitted light when struck by rays from the glass tube. Using the nomenclature for the algebraic unknown ("X"), Roentgen called the mysterious new light "X ray." In the early years, Roentgen and others used X rays to diagnose bone fractures, examine internal organs, and locate foreign objects in tissues. Today, because of scientific advancements in equipment design, *radiology*— a branch of medical science that uses radiant energies—has a far wider scope of application and includes many areas of specialization, such as radiation therapy, nuclear medicine, ultrasound, special procedures, and computed tomography. Figure 1-1 is an overview of areas of specialization in the field of radiography.

Although diversity and specialization exist within the radiological sciences, a core of knowledge and skills is common to all radiographers. Beyond this basic core, there are distinct differences between the scope of practice of a limited radiographer and a radiologic technologist. The differences (educational and scope of practice) between a radiologic technologist and a limited radiographer are readily apparent in the following descriptions.

A *radiologic technologist* has successfully completed a formal educational

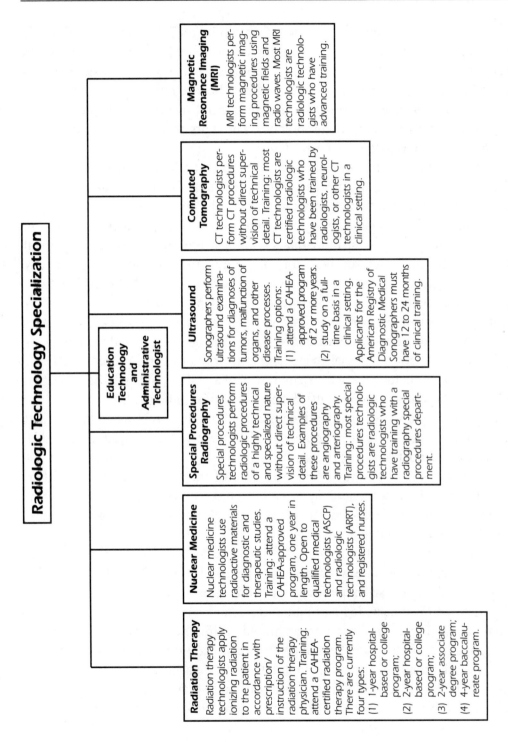

Radiologic Technology Specialization

Radiation Therapy

Radiation therapy technologists apply ionizing radiation to the patient in accordance with prescription/instruction of the radiation therapy physician. Training: attend a CAHEA-certified radiation therapy program. There are currently four types:
(1) 1-year hospital-based or college program;
(2) 2-year hospital-based or college program;
(3) 2-year associate degree program;
(4) 4-year baccalaureate program.

Nuclear Medicine

Nuclear medicine technologists use radioactive materials for diagnostic and therapeutic studies. Training: attend a CAHEA-approved program, one year in length. Open to qualified medical technologists (ASCP) and radiologic technologists (ARRT), and registered nurses.

Special Procedures Radiography

Special procedures technologists perform radiologic procedures of a highly technical and specialized nature without direct supervision of technical detail. Examples of these procedures are angiography and arteriography. Training: most special procedures technologists are radiologic technologists who have training with a radiography special procedures department.

Ultrasound

Sonographers perform ultrasound examinations for diagnoses of tumors, malfunction of organs, and other disease processes. Training options:
(1) attend a CAHEA-approved program of 2 or more years.
(2) study on a full-time basis in a clinical setting.
Applicants for the American Registry of Diagnostic Medical Sonographers must have 12 to 24 months of clinical training.

Computed Tomography

CT technologists perform CT procedures without direct supervision of technical detail. Training: most CT technologists are certified radiologic technologists who have been trained by radiologists, neurologists, or other CT technologists in a clinical setting.

Magnetic Resonance Imaging (MRI)

MRI technologists perform magnetic imaging procedures using magnetic fields and radio waves. Most MRI technologists are radiologic technologists who have advanced training.

Education Technology and Administrative Technologist

Figure 1-1 An overview of specialization in Radiologic Technology

program evaluated by the Joint Review Committee on Education in Radiologic Technology and approved by the Committee on Allied Health Education and Accreditation (CAHEA). Radiologic technologists perform both basic and contrast radiographic procedures as supervised by a licensed practitioner of the healing arts (a person licensed or otherwise authorized to practice medicine, dentistry, podiatry, osteopathy, or chiropractic). These procedures may be performed in hospitals or other medical care settings.

A limited radiographer may have completed formal allied health education in a program such as nursing, medical assisting, medical technology, respiratory therapy, or physical therapy. Such programs generally do not provide radiography education; however, cross training, or a multiskilled approach, is common in medical assisting programs. Individuals coming from allied health educational programs who have not received formal limited radiography education may acquire radiography skills by less traditional methods, such as on-the-job training, correspondence courses, or independent study programs.

A *limited radiographer* performs basic noncontrast radiographic procedures under the supervision of a licensed practitioner of the healing arts. Limited radiographers generally do not perform specialized radiography or fluoroscopic procedures. These procedures often include the use of contrast media and require specific education and training beyond the scope of the duties of a limited radiographer.

Limited radiographers usually are employed in medical offices and outpatient and ambulatory care clinics; in some states, they are also employed in hospitals. A variety of occupational titles exists for workers/staff who perform limited radiography tasks; such titles vary from one area of the United States to another. Thus, the limited radiographer may be called a limited license radiographer, radiographic assistant, limited medical radiographer, practical technologist, or, most recently, limited permittee.

Radiographers may be further classified by state laws that regulate the scope of practice. A number of states recognize ten specific Limited Permittee categories for radiographers: chest, extremities, gastrointestinal, skull, torso-skeletal, dermatology, genito-urinary, leg and podiatric, dental laboratory, and photofluorographic chest. Table 1-1 illustrates geographic differences in occupational titles and regulations. If the reader should desire additional information about classification of radiographers and radiographic tasks in a particular state, contact that state's Radiation Control Office. A listing of such offices may be obtained by contacting The Conference of Radiation Control Program Directors, Inc., 205 Capital Avenue, Frankfort, Kentucky 40601.

Table 1-1 ▪ Limited Medical Radiography Licensure Informational Matrix

STATE	LICENSURE BEGAN	CATEGORIES FOR LIMITED RADIOGRAPHY
Alaska	1971	No regulations or requirements exist for licensure or certification of X-ray operators; however, registrants of medical, dental, or veterinary X-ray equipment are required to (1) assure that all X-ray equipment is operated only by individuals adequately instructed in safe operating procedures and competent in the safe use of equipment, and, (2) provide safety rules to each individual operating X-ray equipment, including any restrictions of the operating technique required for the safe operation of the particular X-ray apparatus, and require that the operator demonstrates familiarity with these rules.
Arizona	1978	Three categories exist: (1) Practical Technologist; (2) Practical Technologist in Radiology (which is limited to chest for lung visualization and Extremities limited to lower two-thirds of humerus and lower distal one-third of femur); (3) Practical Technologist in Podiatry (limited to lower leg below knee). No mandatory CEUs for certification renewal.
California	1971	Ten categories of Limited Permits exist: (1) Chest; (2) Extremities; (3) G.I.; (4) Skull; (5) Torso-Skeletal; (6) Dermatology; (7) G.U.; (8) Leg and Podiatric; (9) Dental Lab; (10) Photofluorographic Chest. California requires twenty-five hours of CEUs every five years. CEU standards are in place.
Colorado	1995	General regulatory provisions related to education and training standards for unlicensed medical personnel exposing patients to ionizing radiation. Those covered include persons at hospital-owned clinics and all other personnel that operate an X-ray machine, i.e., nurses, physician assistants, medical technicians, etc. These persons must successfully complete a limited scope examination specified by their regulatory board, i.e., chiropractic, dental, nursing, podiatry, and veterinary.
Delaware	1987, Amended in 1995	Radiation Technician to include the specific areas of Chest, Extremities, Skull, Spine, Podiatric, and Bone Densitometer.
Florida	1979	Basic X-ray Machine Operator. Persons seeking certification must successfully pass the limited scope examination administered by the American Registry of Radiologic Technologists. Renewal of the basic X-ray machine operator certification requires completion twelve hours of state approved CEUs. Reciprocity may be granted if a person holds a current X-ray certificate or license from another state with requirements that are comparable to those currently in effect.

Table 1-1 ▪ (Continued)

Guam	1997	Currently establishing rules and regulations on radiological protection. These rules and regulations must be approved before implementation of a safety and control program concerning radiation emitting devices.
Hawaii	1978, Repealed in 1995	Provided special temporary permit with general purpose application for chest, abdomen, skull, and extremities as supervised by a radiologic technologist or a licensed practitioner of the healing arts.
Illinois	1984	Three categories: (1) Medical Radiography; (2) Pediatric Radiographic Assistant; (3) Chiropractic Radiographic Assistant. Requires twelve hours of CEUs every year. CEU standards are in place.
Indiana	1981	Five categories of Limited Certification exist: (1) Chest; (2) Podiatry; (3) Dental; (4) Chiropractic; (5) Limited General. Persons must complete formal training and pass an agency approved training program. No mandatory CEUs required for certification renewal every two years.
Iowa	1983	Limited Diagnostic Radiographer in the following five categories: (1) Podiatry; (2) Vertebral Spines; (3) Chest; (4) Extremities; and, (5) Sinus. Requires twelve hours of CEUs every two years. CEU standards in place.
Kentucky	1978	Limited Medical Radiographer (LMR). A person may become certified after satisfactory completion of approved training and passing the limited scope examination administered by the American Registry of Radiologic Technologists. Two training options are available: (1) A state approved limited medical radiography program or, (2) State coordinated limited medical radiography home study program. Twelve hours of CEUs are required to renew the certificate every two years. Reciprocity may be granted if a person holds a current X-ray certificate or license from another state with requirements that are comparable to those currently in effect.
Louisiana	1984	Defines a radiographer as a person, other than a licensed practitioner, who under the direction and supervision of a licensed practitioner applies radiation to humans for diagnostic purposes upon prescription of a licensed practitioner. No personnel shall assume or use the title or designation of "Licensed Radiologic Technologist" unless he or she holds a current license issued to them in accordance with provisions of state regulation. Persons exempt from licensure are: chiropractors' assistants certified by the Louisiana Board of

Table 1-1 ■ (Continued)

		Chiropractic Examiners and persons certified and authorized by the Louisiana State Board of Medical Examiners to perform diagnostic or therapeutic radiological examinations or treatments or both on the premises of the private office of a physician or in a clinic in which a physician practices upon prescription of and under the direction and supervision of a licensed physician.
Maine	1984	Requires persons using ionizing radiation for diagnostic purposes in the office of a licensed practitioner, or physician assistants or nurses to obtain a limited license. In granting a limited license the state approves a course of study, training, and examination applicable to the limited scope of practice of the various disciplines (skull, spine, chest, extremities, and podiatry). Aspects of study, training, and examination relating to patient safety shall be identical to the requirements for a full license. The examination requirement for an applicant who is currently licensed in another state and who possesses a current national certification may be waived. Certificates may be renewed every two years upon completion of twenty-four hours of continuing education.
Maryland	1986	Limited Radiography. Requires thirty hours of CEUs every two years. CEU standards or requirements.
Massachusetts	1988, 1992	Discontinued issuing limited licensure.
Minnesota		The Minnesota Department of Health (MDH) operator examination rule recognizes five examination providers. Persons wishing to receive a certificate from the MDH need to provide proof with evidence of passing one of the applicable radiography examinations. Upon proof of passage, the MDH will issue a certificate acknowledging passage of the examination. No training or education requirements prior to the examination have been imposed.
Montana	1977	Issues a limited practice permit to persons who successfully complete the required formal training (40 hours) and the required examination. The limitations of the permit are as follows: Chest, extremities, spine, skull, abdomen, G.I. tract fluoroscopy. Six hours of CEUs are required to renew the limited practice permit.
Nebraska		Limited system X-ray operator certification. A person may apply for certification upon satisfactory completion of: (1) An approved course of instruction in radiation use and

Table 1-1 ▪ (Continued)

		safety consisting of sixteen hours of instruction and, (2) receive a passing score of 60% on the limited scope examination in radiography administered by the American Registry of Radiologic Technologists. Reciprocity may be granted if a person holds a current certificate as an X-ray system operator or a limited X-ray system operator issued by another state which has the same or comparable certification standards as Nebraska.
New Hampshire		Licensure is required for those performing dental radiography. To qualify for approval to perform dental radiography, the applicant must show evidence of completing a 12 hour course in dental radiography and successful passage of the dental assistant national board examination. Others who perform radiographic examinations on humans must be adequately trained by their employer and must be provided with written instructions for completing the examinations. These persons must be able to demonstrate competency in performing the examinations and may only expose an individual to radiation for healing arts purposes and upon the request of a licensed practitioner of the healing arts. Adequacy of training and demonstration of competence are within the judgment of the employer and not the state.
New Jersey	1969	Provides for licensure of Radiologic Technologists/Diagnostic X-ray (LRT) (R) and limited licensure with specialty categories in the following: (1) Chest X-ray Technologist (LRT) (C), (2) Dental X-ray Technologist (LRT)(D), (3) Radiation Therapy Technologist (LRT)(T), (4) Podiatric X-Ray Technologist (LRT)(P), (5) Orthopedic X-ray Technologist (LRT)(O) and, (6) Urologic X-ray Technologist (LRT)(U). To obtain a license in any limited licensure category, the applicant must meet educational and examination requirements set by the state. Accrual of CEUs is not required for renewal of any limited license category.
New Mexico	1983, 1996	Additional requirements added. A certificate of limited practice is issued to a person practicing procedural radiography, under the supervision of a licensed practitioner or a radiologic technologist, in the areas of: (1) viscera of the thorax, (2) extremities, (3) dentistry, (4) axial/appendicular skeleton; and, (5) foot, ankle, and lower leg. A full certificate is issued to a person who is a radiographer, radiation therapy technologist, or nuclear medi-

Table 1-1 ▪ (Continued)

		cine technologist. To obtain a limited practice certificate, evidence of satisfactory completion of an approved program of didactic and clinical instruction and successful completion of the written examination prescribed by the state for each limited scope specialty for which a certificate of limited practice is requested. Evidence of satisfactory completion of at least twenty hours of approved continuing education is required to renew the limited practice certificate. If a person is qualified in more than one procedure specialty area, it is recommended that CEUs should equalize as closely as possible the education or training in each procedural specialty.
Ohio	1994	Issues a general X-ray machine operator license (GXMO). To obtain a general X-ray machine license, one must satisfactorily complete the required education and an examination identified by the state. Reciprocity is allowed if the individual holds certification in an area of practice from the American Registry of Radiologic Technologists or the American Chiropractic Registry of Radiologic Technologists. If a person obtains a certificate by the "grandfather" clause, they must complete twelve hours of continuing education unless the license holder has already met the educational requirements, then the holder shall complete six classroom hours in topics related to radiation protection specific to the license holders area of practice. Renewal of a general X-ray machine license requires the completion of six hours of CEUs in the area of radiation protection every two years.
Oregon	1979	Provides for the following Limited Permit categories: (1) Skull and Sinuses; (2) Spine; (3) Chest and Ribs; (4) Upper Extremities; (5) Lower Extremities; and (6) Abdomen and Pelvis. Requires twelve hours of CEUs every year. CEU standards are in place.
Pennsylvania	1987*	*On or after January 1, 1988, no auxiliary person may administer radiologic procedures unless the appropriate examination was passed. Two categories of limited radiography: (1) Thorax and Extremities; and, (2) Skull and Sinuses. To obtain certification, one must score 70 or higher on the limited scope examination administered by the American Registry of Radiologic Technologists.

Table 1-1 ▪ (Continued)

South Carolina	1986*	*Effective May 28, 1993 specific regulations were promulgated. Each medical facility is required to ensure that all X-ray operators are adequately instructed in safe operating procedures and competent in the safe use of the equipment. Each operator is required to have instruction, at a minimum, in the following areas: radiation protection, darkroom, machine safety and operation, and general operating procedures. The state evaluates operator training by reviewing the training plan of each facility. Each facility is required to establish a training plan and to document training of each operator in the areas specified above.
Tennessee	1982	Provides for certification of X-ray Operators in the following categories: (1) Chest, (2) Extremity Radiography, (3) Skull (AP and Lateral only), Sinuses, and, (5) Lumbar Spine (AP and Lateral only). Certified operators are required to obtain 20 hours of continuing education credit every two year renewal period.
Texas	1988	Limited Medical Radiologic Technologist Certificates in the following categories: (1) Skull, (2) Chest, (3) Spine, (4) Extremities; (5) Chiropractic, (6) Podiatric, and, (7) Cardiovascular. Persons holding a limited certificate in one or more categories may not perform radiologic procedures involving the use of contrast media, utilization of fluoroscopic equipment, mammography, tomography, bedside radiography, nuclear medicine, and/or radiation therapy procedures. A person holding a limited certificate in the cardiovascular category may perform radiologic procedures involving the use of contrast media and fluoroscopic equipment for the purposes of diagnosing or treating disease or condition of the cardiovascular system. Current licensure or registration as a LMRT by another state whose requirements are more stringent than or substantially equal to the requirements for the Texas limited certificate at the time of application to the state may qualify for an LMRT certificate. Twelve hours of directly related CEUs are required every two year renewal period.
Utah	1990	Certification in practical technician. Persons must pass an examination designated for the limited scope of practice. Requires evidence of 10 hours of CEUs every two year renewal period.

Table 1-1 ▪ (Continued)

Vermont	1978	Limited radiography license in three categories: (1) Chest, (2) Extremities, and, (3) Chest and Extremities. No mandatory CEUs required for license renewal.
Virginia	1997	Radiologic technologist-limited (RTL). A radiologic technologist-limited is permitted to perform radiologic functions within their capabilities and the anatomical limits of their training. An RTL shall not instill contrast media and shall be responsible to a licensed radiologic technologist, doctor of medicine, osteopathy, chiropractic, or podiatry. The RTL license shall be renewed every two years.
Washington		Does not have a limited type of licensure, however, does require registration of X-ray technologists and certification of the following: (1) diagnostic radiologic technologist, (2) therapeutic radiologic technologist, and, (3) nuclear medicine technologist.
Wyoming	1985	Radiologic Technician: A person who has not received formal training but who meets minimum requirements for restricted license. Restricted license provided in specialty category areas of: (1) Skull, (2) Vertebral Spine, (3) Chest, (4) Upper Extremity, (5) Lower Extremity, (6) Pectoral Girdle, and, (7) Podiatric. Requires five hours of CEUs to renew the license every year.

Note: A questionnaire survey was sent to all states to update information provided in this matrix. As of the date of publishing of this revised edition, the following states had not responded to the questionnaire or did not confirm the information as printed. These states are: Alabama, Arkansas, Connecticut, Georgia, Idaho, Kansas, Michigan, Mississippi, Missouri, Nevada, New York, North Carolina, North Dakota, Oklahoma, Rhode Island, South Dakota, West Virginia, Wisconsin.

In 1981, Public Law 97-35 (the Consumer-Patient Radiation Health and Safety Act) was enacted in response to growing concern and awareness about potential long-term effects from radiation exposure.[1] The act gave Congress the power to protect consumers and patients from unnecessary or excessive radiation exposure. To do so, Congress established the following objectives.

1. Provide for the establishment of minimum standards by the federal government for the accreditation of education programs for persons who administer radiologic procedures and for certification of such persons.
2. Ensure that medical and dental radiologic procedures are consistent with rigorous safety precautions and standards.

On 11 December 1985 in the *Federal Register*, the Secretary of Health and Human Services issued 42 CFR Part 75—minimum Standards for Accreditation of Educational Programs For, and the Credentialing of Radiologic Personnel; Final Rule.[2] These standards are intended for use by states in implementing Public Law 97-35.

As of 1989–1990, twenty-six states had complied with or were in the process of complying with the 1981 Consumer-Patient Radiation Safety Act. No sanctions have thus far been imposed upon states that choose to ignore the standards. Refer again to Table 1-1 for an overview of the states that have licensure or certification of limited radiographers.

Philosophy Statement

In its relation to a health care profession, a philosophy statement speaks to the motivating concepts or principles guiding the practice of that profession. Thus, the following philosophy statement of the scope of practice for limited radiography attempts to capture the intent of the Consumer-Patient Radiation Health and Safety Act.

A limited radiographer is a multiskilled person dedicated to assisting in many aspects of medical care. These duties are at the request of and under the supervision of a licensed practitioner of the healing arts. The limited radiographer's scope of practice is confined to radiography of anatomic parts and body regions as regulated by applicable state laws. Although their scope of practice may be confined by law, limited radiographers must have the depth of knowledge and understanding necessary for each radiographic task to assure skill competency and safety as a practitioner. Competence in the occupation also requires that a limited radiographer demonstrate professional characteristics, adhere to ethical and legal standards of medical practice, communicate effectively, and recognize and respond to emergencies to provide maximum protection to the patient.

Occupational Scope and Purpose

Job requirements and responsibilities of a limited radiographer vary from office to office or other practice site; particular qualifications and responsibilities depend upon the medical specialty or geographic area of employment. The scope of duties limited radiographers perform also depends upon applicable state laws. Regardless of these differences, a basic core of knowledge and skills includes the following broad job duty areas:

1. Communication
2. Administrative and clerical functions
3. Patient care and management
4. Support service duties
5. Operation and maintenance of radiographic imaging equipment
6. Operation and maintenance of film processing equipment and supplies
7. Radiation protection
8. Radiographic imaging and patient positioning
9. Radiographic exposure and quality
10. Continuing education

The more experienced limited radiographer may become an office or clinic manager, supervising other personnel and coordinating the overall operations of a medical practice.

Basic to the occupation is the ability and desire to perform as a cooperative member of a medical team. A good perspective from which to view the occupation is to think of it as being "service oriented" rather than "task oriented." The purpose is to function as a medical team member and to help provide quality care for the person undergoing radiographic procedures.

EDUCATION

During the years when limited radiography was beginning to develop as a distinguishable job category, it was a common practice for allied health workers to learn radiography on the job. Of course, some of these individuals had completed formal educational programs in related fields, such as in nursing, medical technology, or medical assisting; however, most of these workers trained in other fields did not have prior education in radiography per se and learned radiographic procedures on the job.

A number of factors, such as consumer awareness of the dangers of radiation and state compliance with the Consumer-Patient Radiation Health and Safety Act, have resulted in the limited radiographer's occupation becoming more than just a series of tasks that can be taught in an on-the-job learning situation. Rather, a structured competency-based educational system is needed to assure that the limited radiographer is a skilled and safe practitioner. A minimum task list is provided in the publication *Task Inventory for Radiography*, available from The American Registry of Radiologic Technologists, 1255 Northland Drive, Mendota Heights, MN 55120.

Many states have adopted the Standards for the Accreditation of Educational Programs for, and the Credentialing of Radiologic Personnel provided by the Department of Health and Human Services, 42 CFR Part 75; December 1985. Implementation of limited radiography training varies from state to state. Some states have developed essentials and guidelines for formal limited radiography educational programs and alternatives—for example, correspondence or independent study programs combined with a supervised on-the-job clinical practicum. In 1987, the Joint Review Committee on Education in Radiologic Technology (JRCERT) "announced that it was studying the question whether a mechanism should be created whereby limited scope of practice educational programs could request evaluation by the JRCERT. The type of recognition that would be awarded is being considered."[3] For further information on the status of the educational standards for a particular state, refer again to Table 1-1.

Limited radiography education may be included with other health occupational programs, such as medical assistant or laboratory technician. Some states have limited radiography education programs designed to admit such individuals as registered nurses or licensed practical or vocational nurses, laboratory technologists, chiropractic or medical assistants, physician assistants, or paramedics. The U.S. Department of Education health occupations newsletter *Lines* (Fall edition 1987) reported that "Several states are planning and implementing programs involving multi-competencies. In Oklahoma, two combinations are being considered (1) combining medical assisting . . . medical laboratory, and radiography and (2) combining radiography, radiation therapy, and sonography."

Figure 1-2 illustrates the cooperation and cross-discipline education occurring between radiology and other allied health professions. The Iowa Administrative Code, Public Health Department [641], rule 42.1 (136 C) states that "licensed practical and registered nurses are permitted to practice as diagnostic radiographers provided they obtain the appropriate training."

Licensed practical and registered nurses are permitted to practice as diagnostic radiographers while under the supervision of a licensed practitioner, provided that the appropriate training standards for use of radiation emitting equipment are met as outlined in the Iowa Administrative Code, Public Health Department [641], rule 42.1 (136 C).

The rules state that the radiation operator must successfully complete an approved 100-hour limited radiography course, such as those offered by the community colleges or the University of Osteopathic Medicine, or a 2-year general radiography curriculum. Upon completion of the course, the nurse must apply for a permit to perform diagnostic radiography from the Iowa Department of Public Health, (515) 281-3478. Within 1 year of completing the course the licensee must pass the state examination for diagnostic radiography.

Radiography continuing education is approved by the Department of Public Health. The continuing education requirements are 12 contact hours per 2 year period for limited radiographers and 24 contact hours per 2 year period for general radiographers.

Either the basic 100-hour limited radiographer course or continuing education may be used for nursing continuing education *IF* the course is also covered by an Iowa Board of Nursing Provider Number. (Ask the providing institution if the course is covered for nurses.)

Any nurse found to be using radiation emitting equipment who has not met the appropriate training standards shall be subject to appropriate proceedings being initiated by the board to determine if probable cause exists for license revocation, suspension, or probation.

Note. Excerpt from *Nursing Newsletter*, Iowa Board of Nursing, 1223 East Court Avenue, Des Moines, IA 50319, November, December 1987, January 1988.

Figure 1-2 Example of cross-discipline education

The Iowa State Board of Nursing also provides for license revocation, suspension, or probation if any nurse is found to be operating radiation equipment without meeting the appropriate training standards.

The American Registry of Radiologic Technologists (ARRT), founded in 1922, has as its purpose the study and elevation of standards of radiologic technology as well as the examining and certifying of eligible candidates. The ARRT recognizes the following disciplines of radiology certification: radiography, nuclear medicine technology, and radiation therapy technology. As of June 1985, the ARRT began to consider the following areas for advanced level examinations: computer imaging, angiography, and magnetic resonance imaging.

In 1983, at the request of several state licensing agencies, the Board of Trustees of the ARRT began to consider the development of examinations covering the tasks performed by an individual having a scope of practice limited to radiography of the chest and/or extremities. The intended purpose of such examinations was for use by licensing states and not for certification by the ARRT.

The first form of the ARRT Examination for Limited Scope of Practice in Radiography (chest/extremities) was administered on 20 March 1986. Not all licensing states have adopted the ARRT examination; several licensing states administer an examination developed by an advisory group of radiologic technology educators. For further information, contact the American Registry of Radiologic Technologists at 1255 Northland Drive, St. Paul, Minnesota 55120-1155.

CONTINUING EDUCATION AND PROFESSIONAL ORGANIZATIONS

Continuing education is encouraged for all allied health professionals and may be obtained by attending professional meetings, seminars, and conventions at county, state, regional, and national levels. Some states have mandatory continuing education policies and require that radiographers show evidence of a certain number of continuing education units (CEUs) in order to renew a certificate or license. Figure 1-3 shows the continuing education sign-in report form used by providers of continuing education units to verify participant attendance.

Continuing education is aimed at improving the quality of work performed by radiographers and increasing their value to the employer and to everyone seeking medical attention. In addition, by taking part in a professional organization, radiographers have an opportunity to develop valuable job networks, enhance technical knowledge and skills, and have a feeling of professional fellowship within the whole occupation of radiology.

SEND TO:
Radiation Operator
  Certification Program
Radiation Control Branch
Bureau for Health Services
275 East Main Street
Frankfort, KY 40601

CONTINUING EDUCATION REPORT FORM
HUMAN RESOURCES/HEALTH SERVICES/RADIATION CONTROL BRANCH
RADIATION OPERATOR CERTIFICATION PROGRAM

NAME	CERTIFICATION NUMBER	SUBJECT TITLE	INSTRUCTOR NAME & TITLE	DATE(S)	HOURS OF INSTRUCTION

Figure 1-3   Kentucky continuing education sign-in report form (adaptation).

Professional growth often results from experiences encountered in the day-to-day medical arena; however, by participating in an organized radiography association, members make a conscious decision about professional growth. The American Society of Radiologic Technologists (ASRT) was established in 1926 and has affiliate societies in each of the fifty states and the Commonwealth of Puerto Rico as well as district groups within the state societies. The ASRT state and district groups provide regular opportunities for radiographers to meet, network and share ideas, hear speakers, and obtain current medical and scientific information.

The national society and some state affiliates publish journals containing timely information for radiographers. Membership in these groups provides continuing education, professional growth, and an opportunity to develop leadership skills. For additional information about the ASRT affiliate in a particular state, contact the national office (American Society of Radiologic Technologists, 15000 Central Avenue, Albuquerque, NM 87123-4605).

OCCUPATIONAL PROGRESS AND PROFESSIONALIZATION

Since 1981, significant progress has been made toward credentialing operators of ionizing radiation equipment and establishing guidelines for educational programs. However, the next decade will determine if limited radiography will be accepted as a vital and necessary level of practice across the United States.

A new profession within radiology may be emerging; the ingredients certainly exist. The following events are signs that professionalization of limited radiography may soon occur:

- The 1981 Consumer-Patient Radiation Health and Safety Act has set forth mandates for training and credentialing.
- The scope and practice of limited radiography has been defined by many states. A task inventory outlining the scope of practice for limited radiographers has been developed by the American Registry of Radiologic Technologists (ARRT).
- Educational training programs have been developed in many states.
- Continuing education is encouraged and required by some states.

These manifestations reflect professional outlook and behavior.

THE FUTURE

It is a certainty that the demand for radiographers will grow in the future. There is also the possibility that the limited radiography scope of practice will increase as the radiologic technologist is called upon to conduct new procedures using sophisticated imaging modalities. As limited radiographers become better educated and more capable, medical professionals may see an opportunity to utilize a multiskilled person.

The future may also bring professional recognition and full acceptance by established radiography associations, accreditation agencies, and other allied health professions. Another future option includes geographic employment flexibility as more states adopt reciprocity guidelines for licensed or certified limited radiographers. Career advancement and mobility are also future possibilities as career ladders, articulation agreements, and competency challenge examinations are developed to allow limited radiographers to advance into radiologic technology and specialized radiography areas.

REVIEW QUESTIONS

1. In a paragraph, describe and discuss the scope and function of a limited radiographer.
2. Compare and contrast the role and function of a limited radiographer to a radiologic technologist.
3. Name the public law that helped to promote educational standards for limited radiographers.
4. List two major objectives of Public Law 97-35, Consumer-Patient Radiation Safety Act.
5. In a paragraph, explain and discuss the importance of lifelong continuing education and professional development for limited radiographers.

REFERENCES

1. Public Law 97-35. Consumer-Patient Radiation Safety Act. Department of Health and Human Services, Public Health Service.
2. 42 CFR Part 75. Standards for the Accreditation of Educational Programs for, and the Credentialing of Radiologic Personnel; Final Rule. *Federal Register*. Vol 50, No. 238, Wednesday, December 11, 1985. Rules and Regulations, 50710-50724. Part II. Department of Health and Human Services, Public Health Service.
3. The American Registry of Radiologic Technologists. *Annual Report*. Minneapolis, MN: The American Registry of Radiologic Technologists, 1987.

Chapter 2

Occupational Standards: Relationships and Communication

Chapter Outline

Objectives

Upon completion of the chapter, the student will meet the following objectives by verifying knowledge, facts, and principles presented through oral and written communication at a level deemed competent and will meet the task objectives by demonstrating the specific behavior as identified in the terminal performance objectives of the procedures.

1. Describe in a written paragraph the importance of positive interpersonal relationships in health care settings.
2. Discuss why there may be differences between how symptomatic and asymptomatic patients perceive the medical environment and suggest ways to avoid miscommunication as a result of these differences.
3. Explain how Abraham Maslow's hierarchy of human needs relates to the radiographer.
4. List three suggestions for creating positive interactions with patients.
5. List and explain five negative barriers to establishing positive relationships.
6. List three suggestions for improving relationships with coworkers, doctors, and supervisors.
7. Describe what is meant by "chain of command" and discuss how it promotes effective communication and team efforts.
8. List five ways the radiographer uses communication in the health care setting.
9. Recall and state an appropriate method of introducing yourself to others.
10. Given sample verbal messages; change them into "I" messages.
11. List five important tips for communicating with referring physicians and agencies.
12. Given sample patient questions, concerns, or statements; use paraphrasing techniques to form a written response.
13. Identify five keys to becoming an effective listener.
14. List five barriers to communication and give suggestions on how to overcome them.
15. Demonstrate competence in each task listed. Refer to the appendix for the individual procedure/performance guides.

    TASKS (See Appendix):

    2-1 Using "I" Messages
    2-2 Using Paraphrasing
    2-3 Using Listening Techniques
    2-4 Recognizing Barriers to Communication

PART I: Relationships

INTRODUCTION

Positive interpersonal relationships are established on a foundation of effective communication, both verbal and nonverbal. This chapter presents suggestions and guidelines for establishing positive relationships with others through effective communication. These guidelines are not intended to be an intimidating list of do's and don'ts, nor are they all inclusive. Rather, they are intended to provide practical suggestions about occupational standards of interpersonal relationships and how to relate to others in health care settings. The limited radiographer should consider these suggestions as only a "starting point," then change and adapt them as needed to specific work situations.

INTERPERSONAL RELATIONSHIPS IN HEALTH CARE SETTINGS

Health care is service oriented and requires constant interaction and communication with others. A limited radiographer's typical day involves talking with patients and their families, doctors, other medical personnel, and people in outside agencies and businesses. One must be able to interact and communicate with a variety of personalities and also be able to observe and listen in order to interpret verbal and nonverbal messages.

Recognizing and responding to the needs of others is a first priority for establishing positive relationships. If the limited radiographer, as well as other members of the health care team, adopts a policy of consumer satisfaction as a daily responsibility, everyone who has contact with the medical facility should have a positive image of the medical facility and staff. In the medical environment, professional image is reflected through individual and group behavior. In today's fast-paced medical setting, one may wonder if projecting a positive image and achieving consumer satisfaction are attainable on a daily basis? Why are these goals a challenge in health care settings? One explanation may be that the nature of the health care environment itself creates a stressful, demanding situation that poses threats and fosters fears, anxieties, and apprehensions.

Interpersonal Relationships with Patients

Limited radiographers generally serve two classifications of patients: those who are not ill or do not have any disease symptoms (*asymptomatic* patients) and those who exhibit disease symptoms (*symptomatic* patients). Asymptomatic patients may be in the medical facility to undergo a routine diagnostic examination. These patients may react and communicate differently from patients who are symptomatic and experiencing pain or discomfort. Differences between patients and their reasons for seeking medical care are key elements in the way patients perceive the medical environment. Most people will have some anxiety, apprehension, and fear of the unknown, yet the degree to which individuals experience these feelings is closely linked to their reason(s) for being a patient. Try to recall or imagine your personal feelings in the following situations:

- You are a patient for an annual checkup. You are in excellent physical condition and feel healthy.
- You are a patient for an examination. You have found a lump in your right breast during self-examination.
- You have smoked one pack of cigarettes every day since you were fourteen years old and have suddenly developed a cough.

The relationship of needs, perceptions, and behaviors can be further explained by considering the hierarchy of human needs.

Hierarchy of Human Needs.   All humans have needs that must be met for both physiological and psychological survival and growth. Physiological needs are related to survival (food, water, air, shelter), whereas psychological needs relate to requirements for love, belonging, and self-esteem. Abraham Maslow, a famous psychologist, described these needs and ranked them in order of importance. Maslow's hierarchy of needs is usually illustrated in a pyramid form with fundamental physiological survival needs having priority over the psychological needs, Figure 2-1.

Maslow believed that people seek to satisfy their physiological needs first. Once these needs are met, people may proceed to fulfill higher-order psychological needs related to emotional and spiritual growth.

Maslow and other psychologists also found that if individuals are confronted with a life-threatening situation, they will defer their psychological needs to only

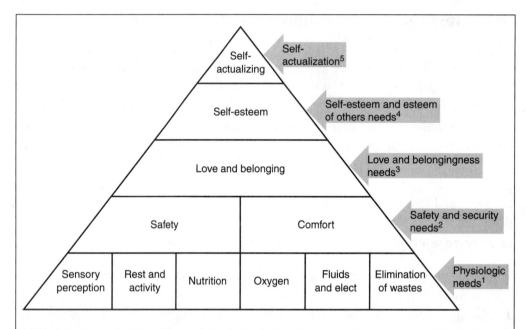

Figure 2-1   Hierarchy of basic needs according to Maslow

1. **Physiologic needs:** Basic life needs for food, shelter, air, water, sleep, and sexual fulfillment. Once these basic needs are satisfied, a person may pursue other needs.

2. **Safety and security needs:** After a person meets his/her physiologic needs, he/she begins to seek a safe place that is sheltered from harm.

3. **Love and belongingness needs:** Once the basic physiologic and safety and security needs are met, the person begins to seek someone to share life and acceptance in a social group.

4. **Self-esteem and the esteem of others needs:** Regard for self comes from positive feedback from others in society. Many emotional and physiological factors impact on self-regard and self-esteem. Before a person can grow and reach a higher level on the pyramid, the lower-level needs must be met and the person must feel a sense of stability and security.

5. **Self-actualization:** After all prior levels of needs have been met, the person begins to grow intellectually and spiritually. Human beings begin to question the nature of life and often seek to fulfill this question by performing humanitarian acts.

those physiologic needs related to survival. This regression or letting go is linked to the primitive survival instinct. In the face of such events, the needs associated with survival generally take precedence over all other needs.

It is important to remember that a person's sense of belonging and feelings of well-being, security, and self-control may be compromised because of an illness. Showing concern—which can be as simple as being courteous—can help in such situations. Using friendly and encouraging words may help others to cope with stressful circumstances. "How are you feeling today?" "May I help you with your coat and umbrella?" "Please," and "Thank you" are all verbal indicators that you want to help and that you value the other person. A smile helps to show caring and a desire to help others.

All people, and especially patients, seek comfort, reassurance, and answers to their questions. They seek to restore balance to their lives by regaining control. Limited radiographers can meet such patient needs by simply taking time to be understanding.

Suggestions for Relating to Patients

- *Show Concern.* Provide a welcome environment. Show concern by being an empathetic, nonjudgmental person. Concern can be expressed by a touch that shows support and encouragement. Don't hurry the patient or appear rushed to get to the next patient.
- *Show Respect.* Showing respect to others is another way of providing a welcome "We Care" environment. All sexes, races, religions, and socioeconomic levels are represented in any patient population. Respect can be verbalized in the way one talks to this diverse population and can be nonverbal via attitude and attention.
- Treat others as you would want to be treated.
- Treat all patients equally regardless of their sex, race, religion, or socioeconomic level.
- Remember children are people too.
- React professionally to what you see or hear while providing patient care.

Respect and concern can be shown by paying attention to detail—"going the extra mile" or "giving one hundred and ten percent" to perform acts of courtesy. Details, often insignificant in a nonmedical environment, can take on great significance when a person is in a threatening or fearful situation. Loss of identity as an individual, Figure 2-2, and lack of privacy can threaten basic human needs. Use the patient's name and provide personal privacy whenever possible.

A person's needs and perceptions can predict the outcome of relationships and communication. Such needs and perceptions influence whether people are open to positive interpersonal relationships or unconsciously set up barriers. Table 2-1 shows positive and negative styles that have such influences.

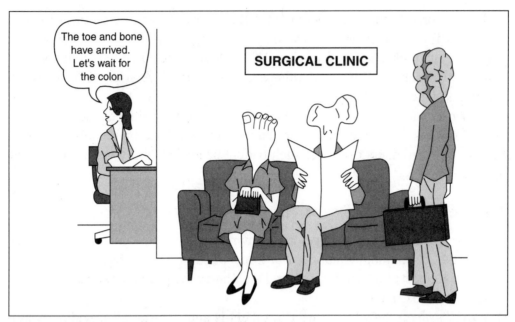

Figure 2-2 Professionals' view of patients. Using patients' names instead of calling them by a number, body part, or procedure shows respect and caring for them as individuals. (*From Purtilo, R. Health Professional/Patient Interactions, 4th ed. Philadelphia: W.B. Saunders Company, 1990, p. 169.*)

Table 2-1 ▪ Establishing Interpersonal Relationships

POSITIVE STYLE (Open to Interpersonal Relationships)	NEGATIVE STYLE (Barriers to Interpersonal Relationships)
Silence	Commanding
Open-ended acknowledgment	Threatening
Listening	Advising
Feedback	Lecturing
Assertiveness	Criticizing
Problem-solving approach	Shaming
	Interpreting
	Sympathizing
	Interrogating
	Humoring

Interpersonal Relationships with Coworkers

Limited radiographers work in settings where many other medical personnel are employed. The entire group of employees is called the health care team. This team should work toward the common goal of providing quality professional services and patient care. It is important that all team members work at peak performance levels and do so in an efficient, cooperative manner. However, in any group of employees there is likely to be some disagreement. Disagreement may occur not only because each team member is an individual with very unique personality traits, but also because health care providers perform their daily duties in a work environment that can be very stressful. How, then, can harmony be achieved? To make the team successful every member must make an effort. Important components of this effort are:

- Effective communication
- Respect for one another
- A positive image about each individual's role as it relates to the entire health care team and to the delivery of professional services.

Frequent staff meetings are one way of allowing everyone to communicate and to refocus the group on the team's objectives. Positive relationships with coworkers do not just happen; rather, they result from behaviors and actions that foster a supportive team feeling. The following behaviors and actions can be used to nurture positive coworker relationships:

- Don't become so preoccupied with work that you forget to extend simple courtesies to your coworkers.
- Prepare a birthday list of all employees, and recognize people on their special day. A cake-and-ice-cream break provides an opportunity for the staff to get together in a nonstressful time period.
- If it is office custom to occasionally bring in doughnuts, take your turn and bring them, even if you don't eat them. What matters is an attitude of "I'm one of you" and "We're in this together." Eating healthy? Bring in a low-fat, low-calorie treat.
- Did you take the last cup of coffee in the pot? Make more coffee.
- If you see a coworker overwhelmed with last minute work, such as filing charts or folding statements, pitch in and help.

- Try eating lunch with coworkers instead of alone. Alone is okay, but it sets you off from the group.
- Adopt a "no gossip" attitude. Positive relationships are built on trust; trust cannot survive in a gossip-filled environment.
- Do you have a problem with a particular person? Try talking with that person about how you feel and see if the problem can be resolved.
- Are you unhappy? You don't like or enjoy being with your coworkers? Consider finding a new job.

Interpersonal Relationships with Physicians and Supervisors

A positive work relationship with physicians and immediate supervisors is important. To reach the medical team's objectives, everyone must be able to communicate effectively and be supportive of each other. This cannot occur when there is disrespect or even dislike for one another.

Suggestions:

- Review the suggestions for positive coworker interpersonal relationships; these also apply to physicians and supervisors.
- Provide positive feedback. Physicians and especially supervisors need to hear that they have done something right or good instead of wrong or bad. If you notice something that physicians or supervisors do that you consider right or good, tell them so. Encouragement and praise can be contagious.
- Address physicians by their title—"Doctor." This helps maintain a professional atmosphere.
- Give and expect common courtesy.
- In conversations with coworkers, patients, or others, reflect an attitude of confidence and support for the physician's professional integrity and ability.

Interpersonal Relationships with Others

Radiographers interact with a variety of people; these include company sales and service representatives, hospital/clinic or medical office staff, service workers, and visitors or patient family members. Everyone should be acknowledged and treated in a pleasant, agreeable manner. Visitors who do not accompany a patient should identify themselves and state the nature of their business.

Generally, sales and service representatives or other business people will present a business card and explain the purpose of their visit. Every medical facility will operate differently, so it is necessary to find out how to greet and handle regular business callers and those who are unsolicited.

The key to effective interpersonal relationships with others is to treat each person as a valuable individual and to treat others as you would like to be treated.

PART II: Communication

INTRODUCTION

In daily life, family members, coworkers, friends, and acquaintances may be able to communicate in loose, imprecise, and familiar ways because the social-personal history between the communicators is known and the circumstances surrounding the message mutually understood. However, in medical care settings, communication must be precise and result in understanding and agreement on what is wrong and what must be done as quickly and accurately as possible. The skill with which communication is accomplished may tilt a delicate relationship or attitude in one crucial direction or another.

CONCEPTS OF COMMUNICATION

Communication may be defined as the exchange of information between two persons. The information is called a *message*. The person who communicates first is the *sender*, and the person to whom the communication is sent is called the *receiver*. The roles of sender and receiver may constantly change during the course of the interchange. This process is one form of communication and the receiver is more likely to interpret the information of the message correctly if the message is simple and precise. The sending and receiving process can become complicated and information misinterpreted because a person's tone, voice modulation, pauses, and nonverbal cues can express attitudes and emotions that the words do not convey. For example, consider the simple message "Close the window." Repeat this message several times, altering your tone of voice, pauses, and body language. Note how methods of expression and tone can confuse understanding of the real message. Imagine how a simple message like "Good morning" can be interpreted if the greeter slams a door immediately after the words are said!

Nonverbal Communication

In this type of communication the message is sent by facial gestures and body motions. A major issue with nonverbal communication is that these messages can be misinterpreted by others. One of the most important nonverbal techniques is eye contact or avoidance of eye contact. In America, looking the other person "straight in the eye" is considered to be the sign of an honest, truthful, sincere person. In Japan, eye contact during a conversation, especially between a subordinate and supervisor, would be considered an insult.

Visual messages, such as facial expressions, are a factor in nonverbal communication and also in self-esteem. For example, facial expressions with a smile and the eyebrows raised can show happiness and offer reassurance; likewise, facial expressions with a frown and the head down can express fear and appear evasive or angry.

In addition to considering appropriate facial expressions for the medical environment, it is necessary to think about the radiographer's general verbal attitude. Is it too casual? Is there too much familiarity with patients or team workers? (e.g., "Hi, Honey" or "Turn over, Honey.") This type of familiarity can embarrass patients undergoing radiography procedures. Socializing with coworkers while performing procedures changes the tone of the encounter.

COMMUNICATION FOR THE LIMITED RADIOGRAPHER

Communication, verbal and nonverbal, is how we present ourselves to others. The combination of what you say, how you say it, and your nonverbal cues while you are saying it form the basis of communication and the impression you make on others. The following are examples of everyday work activities that have such impact:

- Introducing yourself to others
- Giving and receiving messages
- Placing and receiving telephone calls

- Using the intercom system
- Consulting with coworkers, physicians, and supervisors
- Consulting with referring physicians and agencies
- Scheduling patients for radiographs
- Responding to patient concerns, questions, and statements
- Giving patients instructions
- Taking patient information
- Explaining radiographic procedures to patients
- Reporting to coworkers, supervisors, and physicians

A radiographer's most important tool is the ability to really observe what is happening when interacting with others. The words *look*, *hear*, and *feel* are very important when dealing with others. One does not have to ask, "How are you?" Observe the other person's complexion, posture, movement, etc.

Introducing Yourself to Others

In the medical environment, you are like a host or hostess. It is part of your job to greet others and introduce yourself. A usual introduction consists of the verbal exchange and nonthreatening body language.

An example of a verbal exchange is "Hello (Good morning, Good afternoon). I am Susan Spencer." Most facilities require that employees wear a name tag that lists name and job title so patients and others can quickly recall the name.

Body language should vary according to the age (or physical condition) of the person to whom you are introducing yourself. Greet adults face to face with an arm's-length distance between yourself and the other person. Distance is important in communication—if you are too close, you may threaten the other person's private space; if you are too far, you may convey a feeling of unfriendliness. Keep your arms and hands down by your side in a relaxed position. Extend your hand if the other person offers to shake hands. When you greet children, get down to the child's height. This technique can also be used for wheelchair patients.

Taking Messages

Health care providers should always have a pen and pad of paper handy so that oral messages can be written down. Commercial message pads are available that list all the essential parts of a message so a critical part will not be omitted—

time, date, message content, name, and follow-up directions. Tips for writing messages are:

- Write the message.
- Repeat the message you have just written to check the accuracy of its content.
- Relay or act on the message.

Are you forgetful? If so, keep a bulletin board near your work area. Section off a small area and label messages "To Act On." Check this area several times a day.

Talking with Coworkers, Physicians, and Supervisors

Limited radiographers will talk with coworkers, physicians, and supervisors about many things. It is important to remember that if you have a question about a radiography request or any aspect of a procedure, *never* proceed until you seek assistance. There are situations in which the limited radiographer must seek assistance from the supervisor. Knowing when this is necessary comes from recognizing and understanding the chain of command.

A chain of command, formal or informal, exists in every work environment. The physician is usually the leader and may employ a supervisor to direct and manage the health care team. The physician or supervisor leads the team in providing services and meeting objectives. Limited radiographers may be surrounded by authorities who have varying priorities and time-line expectations. The chain of command concept helps address this confusing situation in a positive way by designating one person as supervisor. The supervisor, who knows the overall goals and objectives, focuses the team's efforts on the priorities to be accomplished. For the chain-of-command concept to work and for all team members to be a functioning part of the group, effective communication and relay of information between and among members must be maintained in a systematic way. A chain of command provides a network system and prevents details and important tasks from being overlooked.

If at any time grievances, complaints, or suggestions need to be discussed, the limited radiographer should take these matters to the immediate supervisor. It is okay to have a grievance or complaint, but the chain of command, not an open public arena, should be used to communicate such issues. Employee, coworker,

Table 2-2 ▪ "I" Messages

"YOU" MESSAGE (Blames Others)	"I" MESSAGE (First Part) Describes Feelings	"I" MESSAGE (Second Part) Describes Desired Change
"You really make me mad."	"I'm feeling upset about this."	"I would like to talk with you and see if we can't work this out."

and supervisor communication, if conducted with candor and a problem-solving attitude (identifying what may be unsatisfactory and correcting it if possible), can be very helpful in improving work relationships. This type of interchange tends to identify and solve problems before they become unsolvable.

Using "I" messages is effective when you are giving criticism, explaining a problem, making a suggestion, or expressing an opinion. "I" messages do not make others feel offended or put them in a defensive position. There are two parts to the "I" message: the first part describes your feelings and the second part describes the desired change. The example shown in Table 2-2 illustrates how an "I" message is more effective in communicating a problem than a "You" message.

Talking with Referring Physicians and Agencies

Limited radiographers may have to talk with referring physicians and persons from agencies such as hospitals, nursing homes, or radiology clinics. The following tips should help you perform such tasks efficiently:

- Organize information and questions before contacting the referring physician or agency.
- Gather all facts and needed documents.
- Briefly write down key points.
- Make telephone contact.
- Identify yourself, facility, and reasons for the contact.
- Make notes of necessary information. Review with contact.
- Thank contact for his/her time.
- Chart information if necessary.

Scheduling and Preparation Considerations

Often a patient must be scheduled for multiple X-ray examinations. If contrast media is used, the X-ray examinations must be scheduled in the correct sequence so that residual barium will not be present to obscure anatomic structures of clinical interest. A common rule is: those X-ray examinations whose contrast media is excreted quickly and completely should be scheduled first. The following provides a sequence for scheduling X-ray examinations and those exams that can be performed together.

Sequence: Intravenous Pyleogram (IVP), Gallbladder, Barium Enema, and Upper Gastro-intestinal (UGI)

Exams that can be performed together: Gallbladder and IVP, IVP and Barium Enema, and Gallbladder and G.I.

Responding to Patient Concerns, Questions, and Statements

Limited radiographers are not expected to know all the answers and many times may not be able to release certain information because of confidentiality. However, it is important to always acknowledge patient questions and statements and be perceptive regarding concerns and fears. Effective listening and paraphrasing techniques allow you to respond verbally to patients without appearing curt or that you are withholding the information requested.

Paraphrasing means repeating what a person has said to you but using slightly different words. Paraphrasing a statement helps to determine whether the message has been understood as it was intended, Table 2-3.

Table 2-3 ■ Paraphrasing

PATIENT'S STATEMENT	RADIOGRAPHER'S PARAPHRASE
"You know, when I fell I hit my knee rather hard and it hurts more than the ankle you are X raying."	"Are you saying that your knee hurts as much as your ankle?"

Giving Patient Instructions

Limited radiographers often find themselves giving instructions to patients. These instructions may be as simple as where to find the rest room or as complex as how to take self-administered medication for an outpatient examination. The following tips should help you give patients instructions clearly and accurately:

1. Speak slowly.
2. In case of complex instructions, have a written copy of the instructions for the patient. Instructions you give repeatedly to patients should be printed to save time. This also gives patients a handy reference source if they have questions after they leave the facility.
3. Repeat instructions if necessary.
4. Ask the patient to repeat instructions back to you.
5. Ask for questions. Don't appear hurried. Wait. Answer all questions.
6. Never assume that everyone can read.

Taking Patient Information

Patient information is personal and confidential. Provide for privacy. If you must take patient information in an area where others are waiting, be discreet and use a soft voice. Use simple words and double check information. Often, limited radiographers ask questions of a very personal nature, such as (to a female patient), "Could you be pregnant? When was your last menstrual period?" Avoid an unpleasant communication interchange, keep your voice tone low, move closer to the patient to indicate that a question is private. Go further than just the question. You may want to explain briefly how the question relates to radiographic examinations.

Explaining Radiography Procedures to Patients

Limited radiographers need to be able to explain to the patient the nature of the radiography procedures. This usually consists of simple factual information. After identifying the patient as the correct patient, the radiographer may say, "Hello, my name is Elana Brown. I'm going to take the X rays of your right arm that Dr. Christopher ordered." If the patient shows concern over radiation exposure, you will be able to explain briefly how collimation works and give assurance when you place the protective lead apron across the patient's lap.

If at any time the patient indicates an error, such as "It's not my right arm that needs the X ray, it's my left arm," or refuses to have the X-ray examination, STOP and check with your supervisor or the physician. Never proceed with a radiographic procedure if there is a question about the exact nature of the procedure or if the patient refuses.

Mistakes are often made because of miscommunication. Often, this results from not listening to what others are saying. Listening skills are a critical key to effective communication. Limited radiographers need good listening skills not only when receiving directions from physicians and supervisors but also when gathering information and facts from patients and coworkers. Good listeners do not interrupt when others are talking. Also, good listeners use paraphrasing techniques (see Table 2-3) in order to determine if they understand the message.

Reporting to Coworkers, Physicians, and Supervisors

Limited radiographers and other health care providers may be with a patient longer than the physician is and may detect things that need to be reported. If a patient's condition changes during a radiographic procedure, report the change immediately to the physician. Reporting is usually oral but may require written documentation in the patient record. Reporting tips follow.

- Think first. Be specific. What needs to be reported?
- Report to the appropriate person. (*Never* leave a patient unattended while reporting a change in condition.)

RECOGNIZING COMMON BARRIERS TO COMMUNICATION

Ideally, if everyone recognized common barriers to communication, everyday tasks could be achieved with greater understanding and less effort. However, that is not often the case. Limited radiographers especially need to overcome such barriers, not only when barriers originate in the patient, but also when they are self-initiated. A few common barriers to communication are:

- Poor eye contact
- Interrupting the other person before s/he is finished speaking
- Poor listening skills
  - Thinking ahead instead of listening
  - Pretending to listen
  - Misunderstanding
  - Ignoring what is said
- Poor oral-verbal skills
  - Fear of speaking up
  - Rudely disagreeing
  - Criticizing instead of explaining

REVIEW QUESTIONS

1. In a written paragraph, discuss the following statement. "Positive interpersonal relationships are established on a foundation of effective communication, both verbal and nonverbal."
2. List and discuss two challenges that limited radiographers may encounter in health care settings that create difficulty in maintaining positive interpersonal relationships and effective communication.
3. Compare and contrast the differences that exist in anxiety or apprehension levels between asymptomatic and symptomatic patients.
4. Briefly discuss the physiological and psychological human needs listed in Abraham Maslow's hierarchy of needs as related to the health care setting.
5. Discuss what is meant by this statement: "A person seeks to satisfy the physiological needs and once these are met may proceed to fulfill the higher-order psychological needs."
6. Discuss one patient care situation in which each of the following positive styles may be used: silence, open-ended acknowledgment, listening, feedback, assertiveness, and problem-solving approach.
7. List several suggestions other than those listed in the chapter that may be used to maintain positive work relationships with coworkers, physicians, supervisors, and others.
8. Discuss how facial expressions and body language can create misinterpretation of the oral communication or send a conflicting message.

BIBLIOGRAPHY

Brewner, Margaret M., William C. McMahon, and Michael P. Roche. *Job Survival Skills*. New York: Educational Designs, Inc., 1984.

Chenevert, Melodie. *Special Techniques in Assertiveness Training for Women in the Health Professions*. St. Louis: C.V. Mosby Co., 1978.

Purtilo, Ruth. *Health Professional/Patient Interactions*. 3d ed. Philadelphia: W.B. Saunders Company, 1984.

Chapter 3

Medical Ethics and Law for the Limited Radiographer

Chapter Outline

Objectives

Upon completion of the chapter, the student will meet the following objectives by verifying knowledge of the facts and principles presented through oral and written communication at a level deemed competent.

1. Briefly define professional education according to views based on educational philosophy.
2. Identify criteria of a true profession and the relationship of a true profession to ethics and medical ethics.
3. Briefly define philosophy.
4. Define moral ethics, biomedical ethics, and professional ethics.
5. Differentiate between legal/moral concepts.
6. Define given terms applicable to legal radiography issues.
7. Explain the radiographer's code of ethics.
8. Identify and discuss the AHA Patient's Bill of Rights.
9. Describe certain policies and procedures that must be established for performing radiographic procedures.

INTRODUCTION

In his 1960 book *Patterns of Professional Education*, William McGlothlin identified the major focus of professional education in medicine, nursing, law, teaching, social work, and clinical psychology as direct contact with people—people who are patients, students, or clients and who need help solving their problems.[1] He called these professions, very simply, "helping professions." He said that professional education had two aims: (1) to supply enough professional people to help (quantity) and (2) to assure society that they (professionals) are competent (quality).

McGlothlin's philosophy and definition are not obsolete. In 1983 (23 years later), Edmund Pellegrino, in "What is a Profession?" *Journal of Allied Health*, described true professions as those that deal with humans when they are most vulnerable and when they lack the knowledge to make their own decisions. Thus the professional-patient relationship is not of equal power, because generally all the knowledge is on the side of the professional and the need for help is on the patient's side.[2]

Pellegrino further described true professions as being set apart from sociological structures by philosophical definitions. Relatedly, many occupations that were once regarded as crafts, arts, trades, and commerce have developed many elements associated with traditional professions:

- setting standards for entry
- defining specific skills or knowledge
- establishing educational requirements and curriculum
- forming national organizations
- publishing journals
- setting fees and standards for performance
- setting codes of ethics

All of these elements arise from social accountability. The article points out other elements, however, that constitute higher moral and ethical codes. These evolve from philosophical definitions created by the special nature of human relations when people are vulnerable (sick) and in need. It is clear that the fundamental concepts of health professionals and their ethical education change very little in terms of purpose. Before we consider the philosophy that constitutes medical ethics, let us first look at radiography in the professional perspective.

DEVELOPMENT OF A PROFESSION

Professions deal with people and are bound both by sociological structures and by the need to have a higher moral and ethical code that addresses two additional components: (1) ethics and (2) behavior (or manners). Irvin M. Borish states that a true profession evolves in stages and comes to possess three criteria: (1) developed specialized skills, (2) a humane code of ethics, and (3) ethical respect from society as an honorable vocation.[3]

In light of what Borish holds to be criteria for a true profession, does radiography measure up to the definition? With many clinical specialties, administrators, and educators, radiographers form a highly diverse and specialized group. Compared to some other codes of ethics, the code adopted by the radiography profession is very humane and addresses standards of conduct. With regard to respect from society, does society value radiography as an honorable profession? Do people know who radiographers are and what they do? Who communicates that message? Radiographers must communicate the message, each of us, in whatever role we play—general or limited radiographer, specialist, administrator, or educator. No one else will carry the message for us.

DEFINITIONS OF PHILOSOPHY AND ETHICS

Philosophy

Most of us assume that we practice appropriate behavior and that we understand what ethical behavior is. This is generally true in a society that attempts to philosophically understand all behavior and also attempts to teach that understanding. **Philosophy** deals with the search for truth, the general understanding of values and reality. Many areas are included in philosophy: aesthetics (nature of beauty), epistemology (how knowledge is gained), ethics (what is good and bad; moral duty and obligation), and metaphysics (study of what really exists).

Ethics is the area concerned with the examination of human behavior. There are good and bad behavior and there are times when we are bound by a certain duty or obligation. From the time we are old enough to understand, we begin to learn the difference between right and wrong and that we all are expected to use reasonable care in our behavior toward others.

Ethics

By definition, **ethics** refers to the study of human behavior which involves the study of various cultures, religions, groups, and individuals in a systematic way. It is important to try to understand that all persons who require health care will not have the same attitude toward the health care delivery system.

Biomedical ethics, or **bioethics**, involves the knowledge and application of modern medical technologies. **Professional ethics** relates to standards of conduct, dealing with duties, and the rights and obligations of practitioners. It requires that moral judgments and values be based on reason and that individuals carefully consider and take responsibility for their own actions.

MEDICAL ETHICS

If we consider professional codes of ethics as "a systematic collection of regulations and rules of procedure or conduct"[4] and then think in terms of those members being in the medical profession, we find that many of the rules and regulations are general to all disciplines and specialty areas that comprise the medical profession. Although the following discussion does not pretend to address all the rules or standards relevant to ethical behavior for the health care provider, let us look at several elements relevant to medical ethics.

First, a trusting relationship must be established between the patient and the health care provider (radiographer). Some essential elements in building trust are protecting patients' rights at all times, recognizing the psychological state of patients, realizing that each patient is unique, and exhibiting respect and cooperation in interpersonal relationships with patients and other health care providers.

There are four principles on which trusting relationships are based: (1) autonomy, (2) beneficence, (3) nonmaleficence, and (4) justice.

Autonomy

Autonomy is the freedom to govern self and to make one's own decisions according to one's own moral principles. Individual reasons for actions are personal. If we look at each person as an end in himself/herself, then we see that that person has an inherent right to be respected or treated as an autonomous or self-governing individual. In medical ethics, autonomy is viewed as the right of patients to determine what will be done with their own bodies. Two critical elements that arise out of autonomy are informed consent and confidentiality.

Informed Consent.   This is recognized as an individual's right to autonomy. **Informed consent** means that certain standards of disclosure must be followed to assure a patient's full understanding about a medical procedure or treatment. Standards of disclosure include the following, but may vary with facilities:

1. The patient must receive sufficient information in terms he or she can understand.
2. Details of the procedure or treatment must be outlined and discussed.
3. Potential risks and benefits of the procedure or treatment must be disclosed.
4. All available alternatives must be considered and discussed.

Valid informed consent may be determined when:

1. All information according to standards of disclosure has been adequately communicated.
2. The patient has the capacity to understand all information and can make a fair informed decision.
3. Consent for the treatment or procedure is given voluntarily.

Even though the duty of obtaining an informed consent may be delegated to other trained personnel, the physician who is performing the procedure is ultimately responsible for obtaining and assessing that informed consent has been correctly conducted and completed.

Consent of Minors.   Factors that determine whether a minor's consent to a medical or surgical procedure is legally effective are maturity, age of minor, and emancipation. Consent for performing a procedure on a minor must be obtained from a parent or parents or from someone acting in *loco parentis*, i.e., a supervisor or guardian. Emancipation describes a minor who is married or lives independent of a parent or parents (emancipated from his or her parents). Most states do not require parental consent for medical or surgical procedures if the minor is emancipated.

Mental Capacity.   Generally, a person may not be judged competent for reasons of age, mental illness, debilitating disease, or for any other reason that results in diminished capacity to make a rational decision. A person may be declared legally incompetent through a judicial proceeding and a legal guardian appointed where no legal guardian exists and the physician determines the person to be incompetent. Even though the person may give consent, consent from the spouse or nearest relative should also be obtained.

Implied Consent.   Implied consent is an exception to the rule of informed consent. Implied consent refers to a situation in which a person is unconscious or when a life-threatening emergency exists and no one is available to provide legal permission. It may be assumed in such a situation that because it is an emergency, under normal conditions the patient would give consent to save his or her life or to prevent permanent health impairment. If the patient, however, has previously refused treatment prior to the existence of the situation at issue, implied consent is not valid.

Confidentiality.   Confidentiality is the patient's basic right to privacy. Confidentiality involves legal as well as ethical considerations. Although not deliberate in many cases, confidentiality is generally the most commonly abused aspect of ethics. Health care providers have a tendency to discuss among themselves what they see and hear. However, they are not expected to discuss any disease or condition or its prognosis with the patient or anyone else. If asked such questions by the patient, the radiographer should explain, "I don't know the answer to that, but your doctor will be happy to discuss it with you."

Beneficence and Nonmaleficence

Beneficence relates to duty to others to provide or improve conditions that promote physical and emotional well-being. **Nonmaleficence** refers to preventing or not causing harm intentionally (i.e., physical assault) or not subjecting another to harm. To illustrate how medical decisions sometimes involve issues of beneficence or nonmaleficence, let us consider the medical professional confronted with the situation of a terminally ill patient. Can/should enough drugs to reduce the severity of pain to a comfortable stage be given when, if given, the drugs may hasten death or cause drug addiction? Is it more important that the patient be made comfortable by reducing her/his pain (beneficence) or be put at risk of being harmfully subjected to drug addiction or even early death (nonmaleficence —do no harm)?

Justice

Justice deals with the balancing and fair distribution of medical care, facilities, and resources for society. Simply stated, justice in this sense refers to distributive justice and requires that all economic goods and services be equally distributed unless an unequal distribution would be of greater benefit to all. In some situations, institutions may consider the needs of the poor or those who have less before they consider the needs of more fortunate groups.

LAW FOR THE RADIOGRAPHER

The intent of this chapter is to deal with some legal concepts as they generally apply to health care delivery. To attempt a wide scale, in-depth explanation of the law as it specifically applies to limited radiography in all states would be a major project and beyond the scope of this book. Also, ethical and legal concepts must be situationally applied, according to a particular incident, location, persons involved, and many other elements.

The past several years have seen a steadily increasing need for health care professionals to become knowledgeable about the legal implications of medical practice. In most allied health disciplines, students participating in clinical area learning activities must provide proof of malpractice insurance. Issues relating to malpractice are critical to the health worker. Therefore, it is important to have some general knowledge of the structure of law.

Four Types of Law

There are four types of law: (1) *statutes*, (2) *administrative regulations*, (3) *common law*, and (4) *constitutional law*.

Statutes are laws. They are the principles and rules that are enacted by legislative bodies, such as the Congress of the United States or state legislative bodies. Statutory laws may be amended, expanded, or repealed by the legislative bodies.

Administrative regulations are written by boards or agencies that have been established by legislative bodies for areas where certain kinds of expertise are required to develop specific regulations. Licensing of hospitals, nursing homes, physicians, nurses, and radiographers are some areas where legislators rely on administrative agencies. The regulations are as legally binding as any law the legislators enact.

Common law is a system of applied law and usually develops in the absence of codified written laws or laws enacted through legislation (pertinent statutes). Common law is based on court (i.e., judges') decisions and legal principles and opinion-set precedents considered in those decisions; judges' written opinions often reflect the doctrines of common law. Much common law has evolved over the years and serves to help make decisions in subsequent cases. Common law is legally binding when it is not in conflict with other laws.

Constitutional law is the highest order of law; it is the branch of public law of a nation or state. In matters of constitutional law, the courts do not make law, rather they determine whether a law agrees or is consistent with the constitution of a nation or particular state. If a law is determined to be unconstitutional, it is declared invalid.

Ethical/Legal Behavior

By definition, ethical behavior relates to moral or good conduct, i.e., what is right to do. Legal behavior is what the law or government says we have to do. There are distinctly legal and distinctly moral issues involved in providing medical services. Sometimes what must be done and what should be done become entangled. For example, take the case of a hospital refusing to accept a child who later dies. The hospital had no legal obligation to accept the child, but few people would dispute it may have had a moral obligation to do so. Also consider the case of the physician who has to make the decision to assist or not to assist an injured motorist on the highway.

If the physician decides to assist, he or she assumes the legal obligation of reasonable care and personal liability. However, even under Good Samaritan laws, which vary from state to state, the physician has no legal obligation to assist. The nature or purpose of a Good Samaritan statute is to encourage voluntary medical assistance to strangers in an emergency situation. Thus, the doctor's decision may depend on ethical or moral values. When health care professionals perform their duties, their actions do have an effect on such issues as patients' autonomy, beneficence, nonmaleficence, and justice; because these actions involve moral behavior, they sometimes result in problems that require legal answers.

Professional disciplines, such as radiography, are expected to establish their own moral standards of behavior based on common thinking. In light of so much litigation regarding medical procedures, complex modern medical technology, and patients' rights, the trend is that law is becoming more concretely intermingled with codes of ethics.

Codes of Ethics

Two examples of professional codes of ethics are frequently used to illustrate specific standards of professional conduct: the American Medical Association Principles of Medical Ethics and the American Nurses' Association Code. The American Society of Radiologic Technologists Code of Ethics is another specifically written document, Figure 3-1. All three of these documents are good examples of how aspects of duties, ideals, values, and goals of the professional can be expressed. Historically, professional codes have not been utilized and/or may not have contained appropriate language. Such terms as *fairness*, *justice*, *equality*, *duties*, and *rights* have not been used or their meaning has been only vaguely defined. Written codes of ethics are important because they may help bring about professional autonomy, which is appropriate as long as the intent is to better serve and improve the health care delivery system, not to be self-serving.

Currently, there is no code of ethics specifically written for limited radiographers. It would therefore be prudent for limited radiographers to recognize and follow the existing code of ethics written and adopted by the American Society of Radiologic Technologists.

The Code of Ethics for the Profession of Radiologic Technology was developed and adopted by the American Society of Radiologic Technologists and the American Registry of Radiologic Technologists. As you read the Code of Ethics, you should recognize some areas that reflect the previous discussion on the theory of ethics.

CODE OF ETHICS*

1. The Radiologic Technologist conducts himself/herself in a professional manner, responds to patient needs and supports colleagues and associates in providing quality patient care.

2. The Radiologic Technologist acts to advance the principal objective of the profession to provide services to humanity with full respect for the dignity of mankind.

3. The Radiologic Technologist delivers patient care and service unrestricted by concerns of personal attributes or the nature of the disease or illness, and without discrimination, regardless of sex, race, creed, religion or socioeconomic status.

4. The Radiologic Technologist practices technology founded upon theoretical knowledge and concepts, utilizes equipment and accessories consistent with the purpose for which they have been designed, and employs procedures and techniques appropriately.

5. The Radiologic Technologist assesses situations, exercises care, discretion and judgement, assumes responsibility for professional decisions, and acts in the best interest of the patient.

6. The Radiologic Technologist acts as an agent through observation and communication to obtain pertinent information for the physician to aid in the diagnosis and treatment management of the patient, and recognizes that interpretation and diagnosis are outside the scope of practice for the profession.

7. The Radiologic Technologist utilizes equipment and accessories, employs techniques and procedures, performs services in accordance with an accepted standard of practice, and demonstrates expertise in limiting the radiation exposure to the patient, self and other members of the health care team.

8. The Radiologic Technologist practices ethical conduct appropriate to the profession, and protects the patient's right to quality radiologic technology care.

9. The Radiologic Technologist respects confidences entrusted in the course of professional practice, protects the patient's right to privacy, and reveals confidential information only as required by law or to protect the welfare of the individual or the community.

10. The Radiologic Technologist continually strives to improve knowledge and skills by participating in educational and professional activities, sharing knowledge with colleagues and investigating new and innovative aspects of professional practice. One means available to improve knowledge and skills is through professional continuing education.

---

*Reprinted by permission of the American Society of Radiologic Technologists

Figure 3-1   Code of Ethics

Legal/Ethical Definitions

Before briefly discussing the procedural aspects of radiology, some ethical/ legal definitions pertinent to limited radiographer interaction with patients and limited radiographer/patient relationships need to be clarified.

Assault.   **Assault** is any willful attempt or threat to inflict injury upon the person of another, when coupled with an apparent present ability to do so, and any intentional display of force such as would give the victim reason to fear or expect immediate bodily harm.

Battery.   Battery is any unlawful touching of another which is without justification or excuse.

The ethical concept related to assault and battery is autonomy. Patients must be given full disclosure (informed consent) about what procedure is going to be performed on their bodies. Otherwise, actions toward them could be perceived as intending harm or as touching their bodies without permission.

False Imprisonment.   **False imprisonment** is the conscious restraint of the freedom of another without proper authorization, privilege, or consent of that individual.

The ethical concept related to false imprisonment is again autonomy. No one has the right to physically restrain another against his/her will or without permission. The best approach to immobilizing or restraining a patient who may move during exposure is to discuss the procedure directly with the patient. In the case of children, seek parental permission. The two occasions where restraint is justified are (1) when the patient may pose a physical threat to the limited radiographer and (2) when the patient may pose a physical threat to himself/herself.

Negligence.   **Negligence** is the omission to do something that a reasonable person (guided by those considerations which ordinarily regulate human affairs) would do, or the doing of something which a reasonable and prudent person would not do.

The related ethical concept deals with the basic duty or obligation to do that which is correct or to behave in a reasonable manner. Negligence is probably the most common cause of litigation. But to prove negligence, the plaintiff must establish four facts: (1) that a duty existed, (2) that a duty was breached, (3) that an injury occurred, and (4) that the breach of duty was the proximate cause of the injury. Negligence is usually determined by assessing how something is customarily done by persons (for example, radiographers) in a similar situation performing a similar procedure (radiographic procedures).

Gross Negligence.   **Gross negligence** involves a stronger case of duty. It is intentional failure to perform a manifest duty in reckless disregard of the consequences as affecting the life or property of another.

The related ethical concept is to do no harm, i.e., nonmaleficence. Possibly the strongest determinant for gross negligence is foreseeability. If a situation is clearly a threat or is dangerous to others, and no action is taken to correct the hazard or risk, then one may be held personally accountable for disregard of how others may be affected by a foreseeable hazard.

Defamation.   **Defamation** is the act of bringing harm to another person's reputation through libel (written word) or slander (spoken word).

Defamation is related ethically to confidentiality and is probably the most commonly abused rule of professional conduct. Respecting and protecting the patient's right to privacy (autonomy) is the responsibility of all health care providers. Discussing a patient's medical condition (e.g., AIDS) unnecessarily with another person could be determined as a defamation of character.

Res Ipsa Loquitur.   **Res ipsa loquitur** or "the thing speaks for itself" is a situation where the injured person in no way contributed to her/his injury. That is, the whole incident was under the control of the offender or defendant. Again, negligence becomes obvious.

The ethical concept of nonmaleficence is related to res ipsa loquitur, which is not to cause harm intentionally (negligence) or not to subject another to harm.

PATIENTS' RIGHTS

One of the most important documents to become familiar with in today's health care delivery is the AHA Patient's Bill of Rights, Figure 3-2. The document is based on both the ethical and legal concepts of autonomy and most of its twelve statements deal with confidentiality and informed consent.

PROCEDURAL ASPECTS OF RADIOLOGY

Uppermost in the radiographer's mind is producing not only high-quality diagnostic images but also images of human anatomy that are pleasing to the eye.

A PATIENT'S BILL OF RIGHTS

This policy document presents the official position of the American Hospital Association as approved by the Board of Trustees and House of Delegates.

The American Hospital Association presents a Patient's Bill of Rights with the expectation that observance of these rights will contribute to more effective patient care and greater satisfaction for the patient, his physician, and the hospital organization. Further, the Association presents these rights in the expectation that they will be supported by the hospital on behalf of its patients, as an integral part of the healing process. It is recognized that a personal relationship between the physician and the patient is essential for the provision of proper medical care. The traditional physician-patient relationship takes on a new dimension when care is rendered within an organizational structure. Legal precedent has established that the institution itself also has a responsibility to the patient. It is in recognition of these factors that these rights are affirmed.

1. The patient has the right to considerate and respectful care.
2. The patient has the right to obtain from his physician complete current information concerning his diagnosis, treatment, and prognosis in terms the patient can be reasonably expected to understand. When it is not medically advisable to give such information to the patient, the information should be made available to an appropriate person in his behalf. He has the right to know, by name, the physician responsible for coordinating his care.
3. The patient has the right to receive from his physician information necessary to give informed consent prior to the start of any procedure and/or treatment. Except in emergencies, such information for informed consent should include but not necessarily be limited to the specific procedure and/or treatment, the medically significant risks involved, and the probable duration of incapacitation. Where medically significant alternatives for care or treatment exist, or when the patient requests information concerning medical alternatives, the patient has the right to such information. The patient also has the right to know the name of the person responsible for the procedures and/or treatment.
4. The patient has the right to refuse treatment to the extent permitted by law and to be informed of the medical consequences of his action.
5. The patient has the right to every consideration of his privacy concerning his own medical care program. Case discussion, consultation, examination, and treatment are confidential and should be conducted discreetly. Those not directly involved in his care must have the permission of the patient to be present.

continues

Figure 3-2 A Patient's Bill of Rights *(Reprinted with permission of the American Hospital Association, Copyright 1992).*

6. The patient has the right to expect that all communications and records pertaining to his care should be treated as confidential.

7. The patient has the right to expect that within its capacity a hospital must make reasonable response to the request of a patient for services. The hospital must provide evaluation, service, and/or referral as indicated by the urgency of the case. When medically permissible, a patient may be transferred to another facility only after he has received complete information and explanation concerning the needs for and alternatives to such a transfer. The institution to which the patient is to be transferred must first have accepted the patient for transfer.

8. The patient has the right to obtain information as to any relationship of his hospital to other health care and educational institutions insofar as his care is concerned. The patient has the right to obtain information as to the existence of any professional relationships among individuals, by name, who are treating him.

9. The patient has the right to be advised if the hospital proposes to engage in or perform human experimentation affecting his care or treatment. The patient has the right to refuse to participate in such research projects.

10. The patient has the right to expect reasonable continuity of care. He has the right to know in advance what appointment times and physicians are available and where. The patient has the right to expect that the hospital will provide a mechanism whereby he is informed by his physician or a delegate of the physician of the patient's continuing health care requirements following discharge.

11. The patient has the right to examine and receive an explanation of his bill regardless of source of payment.

12. The patient has the right to know what hospital rules and regulations apply to his conduct as a patient.

No catalog of rights can guarantee for the patient the kind of treatment he has a right to expect. A hospital has many functions to perform, including the prevention and treatment of disease, the education of both health professionals and patients, and the conduct of clinical research. All these activities must be conducted with an overriding concern for the patient, and, above all, the recognition of his dignity as a human being. Success in achieving this recognition assures success in the defense of the rights of the patient.

Figure 3-2 *continued*

However, we must take all aspects of the finished radiograph into consideration. Although not limited to this discussion, some of the most important aspects deal with how we produce a radiograph from beginning to end and what could happen during the performance relevant to (1) the examination request, (2) film labeling, (3) film identification, (4) records, (5) retention of records, (6) informed consent forms, (7) radiation safety, (8) equipment safety (refer to compliance regulations and technologist certification), and (9) procedure complications. Some of these elements have relevance to our discussion in the earlier part of the chapter, particularly some elements related to autonomy (informed consent and confidentiality), beneficence, and nonmaleficence.

Examination Request

Before ever seeing the patient, the radiographer receives an examination request that has been written by the patient's attending physician. Items included on the requisition include the patient's name and vital statistics, the type of radiographic procedure to be performed (e.g., chest), why it needs to be done (history), and the doctor's signature.

A common practice is for the radiographer to ask the female patient who is of appropriate (childbearing) age when she had her last menstrual period (LMP). The information should be written on the request; some practitioners prefer to have the patient's personal signature in the LMP area of request. Where this is the policy and a patient is unable to sign her name, the attending physician or a guardian may sign for her.

The limited radiographer is clearly placed in a decision-making position when reading the examination request (1) to make sure signatures are appropriate, (2) to assure that critical questions have been asked, and (3) to determine that the patient's medical history relating to the radiographic examination is written on the request. The information included on an examination request is critical to making sure that the proper examination is done and that the radiologist has sufficient background information to aid in interpreting the radiographic image. Although examination requests are more commonly computer-generated in most radiology office and hospital departments, an example is included in Figure 3-3.

APPT. #	CURR. X-RAY #	NAME		TODAY'S DATE	TIME	PAGE

BIRTH DATE	AGE	M/F	HOSPITAL #	EMER. REC. #	

ADDRESS 1		ADDRESS 2		CITY	STATE	ZIP

HOME PHONE	WORK PHONE	HOSP. ROOM	BED	SCHED. BY	CHANGED BY

REFERRING PHYSICIAN 1	REFERRING PHYSICIAN 2

RADIOLOGIST	10E	TRANSPORT	ADMITTING DIAGNOSIS

APPOINTMENT REMARKS	PREGNANT	LMP	DEPARTMENT	

SPECIAL HANDLING

TECH	# FILMS	FILM TYPE	TECH NOTES

PAT RQST	PAT ARVL	EXAM START	EXAM END	LEFT DEPT

PREVIOUS EXAMS

Figure 3-3 Radiographic examination request

Film Labeling/Identification

Film labeling, using lead letters to indicate the patient's identification and that the correct side of the body has been marked, is crucial. If a film has no markings on it, it really belongs to no one and therefore has no value and should be discarded. If for some reason, a film was not labeled at the time it was taken, it must be marked immediately after processing. Legally, the markings should be put on the film in a permanent manner (e.g., a black felt pen). This shows there was no intent of deception and that the one who marked the film can demonstrate that the markings are clearly correct.

Radiographs as Permanent Records

Radiographs are permanent records. Although the information contained in records is subject to the patient's use, the records belong to the office or institution where they were made. It is therefore important that these records be accurately maintained for future purposes. Some important reasons are: (1) follow-up for certain diseases or conditions, e.g., cancer, emphysema; (2) annual physical, e.g., chest examinations; (3) legal procedures, such as in trauma cases; and (4) research and teaching. Appropriate policies and procedures must be established for not losing films when they are loaned to doctors or other persons (i.e., lawyers). There also must be policies established regarding films subpoenaed for litigation. These kinds of policies are a protection for everyone involved. (See sample release form, Figure 3-4.)

Releasing Films

The following procedures are suggested for releasing films from the office or department to other physicians, the patient, or other than medical personnel.

1. *Other physicians*—a release form must be filled out by the patient. The films may be transferred to a different film jacket to be sent out. (Until the films are returned, the original film jacket and reports are refiled.) The jacket for sending out should be stamped *Please Return* to with your office name and address provided (like a self-addressed reply envelope).
2. *The patient*—the patient must fill out a release form and sign it. The doctor to whom the patient is taking the film should be notified. When the films have served the intended purpose, they must be returned to the proper office or department.

REQUEST FOR RELEASE OF RADIOGRAPHIC FILM

Request is made by the undersigned patient to review personal radiographic films on file at _____ Hospital/Clinic.

_____
DATE

_____
SIGNATURE OF PATIENT

PATIENT'S SS#_____

_____
SIGNATURE OF PERSON AUTHORIZING RELEASE

Film Record Room Information:

_____
PATIENT'S NAME (PRINTED)

_____
SIGNATURE OF RADIOLOGIST

FILM REPORT INCLUDED: YES _____   NO _____

PURPOSE OF RELEASE _____

_____

_____
DATE REMOVED

_____
PERSON RELEASING

_____
DATE RETURNED

Figure 3-4   Sample release form

3. *Other than medical personnel*—this category includes such persons as lawyers and insurance company personnel. A release/consent form must be filled out by the patient and/or the physician. Generally, a fee is charged to attorneys or insurance agencies for release of a patient's film.

The best method for record keeping today is through computerized programs so that standard procedures and accuracy may be ensured. The length of time that medical records must be kept depends on state regulations regarding medical records. Generally five years of current films are kept in files and then purged for storage or discard. If films are of minors, the length of time they must be kept may be longer than five years. Radiology records also provide information for administrative reports. A daily log of appointments and procedures is generally maintained; billing is indicated for examinations completed. Quality control reports are generated to show film usage and numbers and types of procedures completed.

Informed Consent Forms

Informed consent forms must always be available and limited radiographers must be educated in their appropriate use. Informed consents should be written so that persons from all levels of education may understand them. The forms should indicate that the patient has been appropriately informed about the risks, benefits, and alternatives with regard to the procedure to be performed on the patient's body. If the duty has been delegated by the physician, the limited radiographer should make sure the consent form has been signed and is in the patient's record for review by the physician prior to doing the radiographic procedure. If the form is not appropriately completed, medical personnel and the office or institution involved in performing the procedure may be subject to legal action should any mistakes or unexpected events occur. (See sample consent form, Figure 3-5.)

Radiation Safety

Radiation safety must be in compliance with (1) the National Council on Radiation Protection and Measurements (NCRP), which is a regulatory agency for evaluating the relationship between radiation exposure and biological effects; and (2) the Consumer-Patient Radiation Health and Safety Act of 1981 (refer to chapter 1), which deals with the establishment of minimum standards for accreditation of radiologic technology programs for persons who administer radiographic procedures. Radiation safety procedures must be written and documentation of equipment inspections must be kept on file at the office or facility.

PATIENT'S CONSENT STATEMENT FOR RADIOGRAPHIC PROCEDURE

I, _____, understand that my doctor, _____

(physician performing procedure)

has ordered a _____ which requires the injection or introduction of

(type of procedure)

_____ into my body for diagnostic purposes.

(contrast medium)

I have answered the following questions as far as I know them to be true according to my personal knowledge.

Are you allergic to any types of: medication ☐   food ☐   shellfish ☐   other ☐

If so, what? _____

_____

Have you ever had any of the following? (Check all that apply)

☐ Asthma	☐ Diabetes	☐ Neurological Problems
☐ Cardiac (Heart) Disease	☐ Renal (Kidney) Disease	☐ Do not know

If you have had this radiographic procedure before or any similar type procedure that included an injection, did you have any problems after the injection?

_____

_____

After reading and discussing this form, and having my questions answered satisfactorily by the physician performing the procedure, I voluntarily consent to the injection of contrast medium for the following procedure: _____

_____   Date: _____

(Signature of Patient)

Witness: _____

Patient is unable to consent because: _____

_____

_____   Date: _____

(Signature of legal guardian or
closest available relative)

Witness: _____   Witness: _____

_____

Note. This is a sample only. Consent forms are designed for specific use and must be checked with legal counsel before use. Consent forms should be obtained by the performing physician or other qualified persons trained in managing such procedures.

Figure 3-5   Radiographic informed consent form

REVIEW QUESTIONS ━━━━━━━━━━━━━━━━━━━━

1. Ethics is concerned with
   a) nature of beauty
   b) what really exists
   c) human behavior
   d) knowledge gained

2. Professional ethics relates to
   a) modern technology
   b) standards of conduct
   c) metaphysics
   d) truth

3. The freedom to govern self is based on
   a) justice
   b) autonomy
   c) confidentiality
   d) beneficence

4. The person legally responsible for obtaining and assessing correct informed consent is the
   a) limited radiographer
   b) patient
   c) physician performing the procedure
   d) referring physician

5. The patient's basic right to privacy is based on
   a) type of illness
   b) informed decision
   c) confidentiality
   d) beneficence

6. Nonmaleficence refers to
   a) disclosing information
   b) doing duty toward others
   c) distributing fairly
   d) doing no harm

7. Principles and rules enacted by legislative bodies are
   a) common law
   b) statutes
   c) administrative regulations
   d) none of the above

8. Fairness, justice, duties, rights, and equality are terms that should be used to develop
   a) administrative regulations
   b) disclosure of information
   c) codes of ethics
   d) all of the above

9. Unlawful touching of another without permission is
   a) battery
   b) assault
   c) negligence
   d) false imprisonment

10. Conscious restraint of freedom is
    a) negligence
    b) defamation
    c) false imprisonment
    d) battery

11. True professionals are said to be individuals involved in human relations in health care delivery, drafts, trades, and commerce.
    a) true
    b) false

12. True professions deal with humans when they are vulnerable; thus, practitioners of those professions are held to a higher standard of conduct.
    a) true
    b) false

13. A true profession may be associated with the following element(s)
    a) humane codes of ethics
    b) specialized skills
    c) society's respect as an honorable vocation
    d) a and b only
    e) a, b, and c

14. There are four general types of law.
    a) true
    b) false

15. Administrative regulations that are written by agencies or boards established by legislative bodies are as legally binding as statutes.
    a) true
    b) false

16. The patient's bill of rights is based on
    a) autonomy
    b) informed consent
    c) confidentiality
    d) a and c
    e) a, b, and c

17. Unmarked films that are marked after processing may be marked with a black marker so long as there is no apparent intent of deception and the radiographer who produced the films can demonstrate that the markings are clearly correct.
    a) true
    b) false

18. Radiographs as permanent records belong to the
    a) patient
    b) physician's office
    c) hospital
    d) b and c
    e) a, b, and c

19. Films may be released under specific conditions to the following
    a) other physicians
    b) the patient
    c) lawyers and insurance companies
    d) a and c
    e) a, b, and c

20. The regulatory agency established for evaluation of the relationship between radiation exposure and biological effects is
    a) Consumer-Patient Health and Safety Act 1981
    b) National Council on Radiation Protection and Measurements
    c) a and b
    d) none of the above

REFERENCES

1. McGlothlin, William. *Patterns of Professional Education*. New York: Putnam, 1960.
2. Pellegrino, Edmund. "What Is A Profession?" *Journal of Allied Health* 12, no. 3 (1983).
3. Borish, Irvin M. "The Academy and Professionalism," *The American Journal of Optometry & Physiological Optics*, 1983.
4. *The American Heritage Dictionary* (2d College Edition). Boston: Houghton Mifflin Company, 1991, p. 287.

BIBLIOGRAPHY

Engelhardt, H. Tristram Jr. *The Foundations of Bioethics*. 2nd ed. New York: Oxford University Press, 1996.

Obergfell, Ann. *Law and Ethics in Diagnostic Imaging and Therapeutic Radiology*. Philadelphia: W. B. Saunders Company, 1995.

Pozgar, George D. *Legal Aspects of Health Care Administration*. 6th ed. Rockville, MD: Aspen Publications, 1996.

Veatch, Robert M. and Harley S. Flack. *Case Studies in Allied Health Ethics*. Upper Saddle River, NJ: Prentice Hall.

Veatch, Robert M. *Medical Ethics*. 2nd ed. Boston: Jones and Bartlett Publishers.

Weston, Anthony. *A Practical Companion to Ethics*. New York: Oxford University Press, 1977.

Wilson, Bettye G. *Ethics and Basic Law for Medical Imaging Professionals*. Philadelphia: F. A. Davis Company.

Chapter 4

Medical Asepsis and Patient Care

Chapter Outline

Meeting Patients' Needs
  Physical Needs
  Other Needs
IV Tubes, Urinary Catheters, Nasal Oxygen
Vital Signs
  Temperature
  Pulse
  Respiration
  Blood Pressure
Medical Emergencies
  Medical Emergencies Terminology
  Fainting
  Seizures
  Vomiting
  Nosebleeds
  Fractures and Spinal Injuries

Objectives

Upon completion of the chapter, the student will meet the following objectives by verifying knowledge, facts, and principles presented through oral and written communication at a level deemed competent and will meet the task objectives by demonstrating the specific behavior as identified in the terminal performance objectives of the procedures.

1. Describe the limited radiographer's role in preventing the spread of microorganisms.

2. Recall and outline the requirements for microbial growth.

3. Differentiate between the levels of infection control by comparing and contrasting methods and uses of medical asepsis, disinfection, and surgical asepsis.

4. Recall the Centers for Disease Control and Prevention's recommendations for prevention of HIV, hepatitis B, and other communicable diseases.

5. Identify common safety measures that the limited radiographer can practice.

6. Identify principles of body mechanics and relate these to radiographer and patient safety and comfort.

7. Identify the common vital signs and describe their importance in the assessment of patient conditions.

8. Identify normal vital sign ranges for adults and children, to include temperature, pulse, respiration, and blood pressure.

9. Discriminate between appropriate and inappropriate procedures and techniques related to taking and recording vital signs, administering oxygen, responding to emergencies, and handling trauma patients.

10. Define what constitutes a medical emergency and identify the limited radiographer's role.

11. Demonstrate competence in each task listed below. Refer to the appendix for the individual procedure/performance guides.

TASKS (See Appendix):

4-1 Hand Washing
4-2 Assisting the Falling Patient
4-3 Preparing Safety Reports (Accident/Incident)
4-4 Using a Three-Carrier Lift to Transfer the Patient
4-5 Transferring a Patient Using a Sheet
4-6 Logrolling the Patient
4-7 Assisting the Patient with Ambulatory Aid: Cane, Walker, and Crutches
4-8 Transporting the Patient in a Wheelchair
4-9 Transferring the Patient between Radiographic Table and Wheelchair
4-10 Preparing Patient for Radiographic Examination
4-11 Taking Temperature by Mercury, Electronic, and Tympanic Thermometer
4-12 Counting the Radial Pulse and Respiratory Rate
4-13 Taking Blood Pressure

INTRODUCTION

Today, health care is provided in a variety of settings, from hospitals offering a wide range of services to those providing specialized care, such as community health agencies, private medical offices, mobile van care units, ambulatory emergency clinics, nursing homes, hospices, and self-help organizations. Home health care is becoming a vital service in the health care industry; so are health maintenance organizations, which stress a holistic wellness approach. Rehabilitation is also very important today to help people return to an active life after an accident or illness.

The traditional objectives of medical science—prevention, detection, and treatment of disease—remain the foundations for delivery of health care. However, ethical, moral, and legal debates are taking issue with procedures used to initiate, prolong, and redesign the life process. As scientific advances continue to expand the role and scope of health care, these and other ethical and legal questions concerning rights and responsibilities will continue to be addressed.

Despite these unanswered questions and the turmoil they bring to the entire health care community, the everyday needs of patients seeking health care must be served. The limited radiographer's primary responsibility is to provide diagnostic-quality radiographs as requested by a licensed practitioner of the healing arts. Because of the nature of the work, limited radiographers also give basic patient care and have an important role in the entire process of health care delivery.

INFECTION CONTROL

Medical institutions, clinics, doctors' offices, and others provide services to many people. **Infection control**, i.e., the prevention of the spread of infectious conditions and diseases, is an important responsibility and goal for everyone. Consider the unlimited possibilities for disease transmission and cross infection between and among the many people who enter a medical facility. Infection can spread from a single focal point or person of contamination to many other parts of the medical care chain and the general public, Figure 4-1.

Limited radiographers are responsible for preventing the spread of micro-organisms to others and for protecting themselves from contamination. By consistent application of basic techniques of hand washing, proper disinfection, and disposal of contaminated items, the total number of infectious organisms can be reduced or diluted to a harmless level.

The goal then becomes to protect self, patient, and others from becoming infected and from serving as a source of infectious organisms to others.

MICROORGANISMS

The environment is teeming with **microorganisms**, which are extremely small and invisible except by microscope. Microorganisms also reside on all skin surfaces of the body and are especially numerous in the respiratory passages, mouth, and entire length of the digestive system. Not all microorganisms are harmful; microorganisms that are not harmful are called **nonpathogenic**. Those that are harmful and capable of causing diseases are referred to as **germs** or **pathogenic organisms**. The five general classifications of microorganisms are *bacteria, fungi, protozoa, rickettsiae*, and *viruses*.

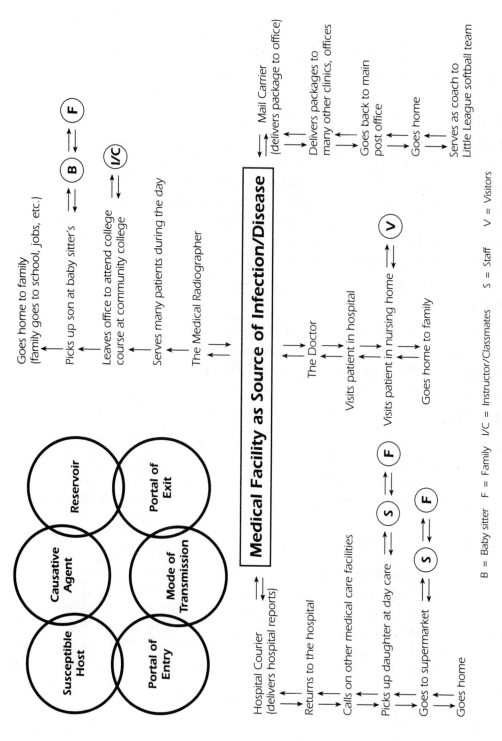

Figure 4-1 Cycle of infection

Bacteria

Bacteria are one-celled organisms, both pathogenic and nonpathogenic, and are identified and classified according to their morphology (shape) and structure.

Fungi

Fungi exist in two forms, yeasts and molds. Yeasts are one-celled animals, whereas molds are multicelled. Approximately fifty percent of all fungi may cause disease in humans. Fungi require moisture and darkness to survive and are often called opportunistic because they are not particularly pathogenic until they encounter a compromised host. Fungi infections occur under numerous conditions and may be a symptom of a more serious disease or infection. Common fungal diseases are thrush, moniliasis, and histoplasmosis.

Protozoa

Protozoa are microscopic one-celled animals. Infection occurs as a result of ingestion of the parasite or from an insect/animal bite. Examples of protozoal diseases are amebiasis, malaria, and toxoplasmosis.

Rickettsiae

Rickettsiae are microscopic life forms found in tissues of fleas, lice, ticks, and other insects. Rickettsial infections are transmitted to humans by the bite of infected insects, which are called a **vector** or the carrier of disease. Common examples of rickettsial diseases are typhus and Rocky Mountain spotted fever.

Viruses

Viruses are the smallest known organisms. Viruses cannot exist outside a living cell and can only be seen by means of the electron microscope. Humans are susceptible to several hundred different viruses. Common virus infections are influenza, measles, German measles, mumps, chicken pox, herpes simplex, and smallpox. Because of their prevalence, viruses are an important consideration in infection control. They are spread primarily by humans via respiratory and intestinal excretions.

NOSOCOMIAL INFECTIONS

Nosocomial infections are often called opportunistic infections. The term is used to describe a group of infections caused by resistant and extremely pathogenic bacteria. These infections occur in hospitals and medical care settings and cause wound, urinary, and upper respiratory infections. They are considered opportunistic since they are more likely to occur in persons with weakened immune defenses due to injury, disease, or long-term antibiotic or corticosteroid drug use. Common opportunistic infections are caused by *Staphylococcus* bacteria ("Staph"), *Escherichia coli*, and *pseudomonas aeruginosa*. Nosocomial infections are spread more by hands than any other method, so proper hand washing can reduce their spread.

MICROBIAL GROWTH AND INFECTION

Microorganisms have certain specific requirements for growth. Knowing these requirements will help the radiographer recognize and eliminate conditions conducive to microbial growth. In this way, the spread of infection to others can be inhibited.

REQUIREMENTS FOR GROWTH:
1. **Host** or reservoir in which to live and grow. The host can be a human being, animal, soil, water, or food. Hosts must provide water and nourishment for the microorganisms.
2. Warm and dark environment. Most microorganisms grow best at body temperature (98.6 degrees Fahrenheit) and prefer a dark environment.

Microorganisms can be spread by a number of methods, Figure 4-2. Infection is caused when microorganisms enter a susceptible host and grow in the body. An infection can be localized or affect the entire body. The factors involved in the process of infection are:

- source of infection (reservoir)
- the microorganisms (causative agent)
- a portal of exit from the reservoir
- a host with a level of susceptibility and a portal of entry

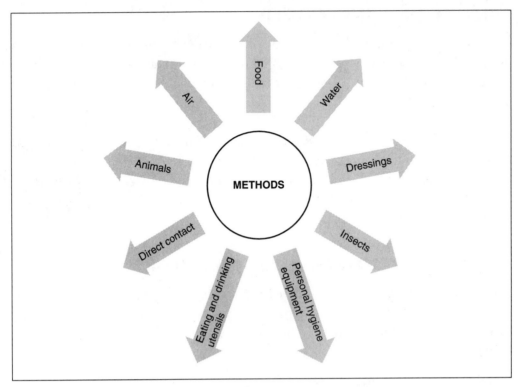

Figure 4-2   Methods of spreading microorganisms

Direct spread of microorganisms occurs when the microorganisms are passed from one person to another by touching or contact. Indirect spread of microorganisms involves the transmission of pathogens by one of three means:

1. Fomites: A **fomite** is an object that has been contaminated with the pathogen. Common examples are a limited radiographer's uniform or the radiographic table. Common fomites are doors, examination tables, equipment, and hypodermic needles.
2. Vector: A **vector** is an animal or insect whose body serves as host to the pathogen. The bite of the infected vector spreads the disease.

Disease	*Vector*
Rabies	Bats, dogs, etc.
Bubonic Plague	Fleas
Rat bite fevers	Rats
Malaria	Mosquitoes

3. Airborne: **Airborne pathogens** are spread by dust or droplet contamination. This occurs when infected individuals sneeze or cough toward a susceptible host.

Remember the following important facts about microorganisms as they relate to the spread of infection:

- Microorganisms are everywhere in our environment.
- Microorganisms cannot move by themselves, but must be transported from one host to another.
- Microorganisms are opportunistic.
- Severity of infection depends on:
    number of pathogenic organisms present
    virulence (strength) of organisms
    resistance of infected person

The human body's defenses are usually strong enough to protect against invading opportunistic microorganisms. However, those seeking health care may have a medical condition or a compromised immune system that leaves them with reduced defenses against the attack.

LEVELS OF INFECTION CONTROL

Infection control includes various actions and procedures that reduce or eliminate the number of pathogenic organisms present. There are three levels of infection control: asepsis, disinfection, and surgical asepsis.

Asepsis

Asepsis is defined as the absence of all disease-producing microorganisms and is very important to breaking the infection cycle. Aseptic techniques physically eliminate pathogens and the conditions that promote their growth and spread. Such techniques include proper hand washing, handling and disposing of contaminated linens, and housekeeping.

Hand Washing.   The hands are a limited radiographer's tools. Radiographers constantly use their hands to prepare the examination room and equipment, to assist and position the patient, and to perform all the tasks associated with providing radiographs. During these tasks, the hands are exposed to pathogens that can infect the limited radiographer, who, in turn, can become a reservoir of infection passed on to others. For this reason, individuals providing medical care should not wear rings (except for a simple wedding band) or have chipped nail polish because these may be contaminated by pathogenic microorganisms.

To prevent the spread of infectious microorganisms hands must be washed frequently, such as before and after working with each patient. It may be necessary to wash hands several times during the period of patient contact for a specific radiographic procedure. In addition to frequent hand washing, any cut or break in the skin should be covered with a sterile dressing. Since dry, chapped, or abraded skin also serves as a portal of entry for microorganisms, care should be taken to keep the skin smooth and intact. **Refer to Task 4-1 in the Appendix for the hand washing procedure.**

Handling and Disposing of Linens.   All used linen should be considered soiled and a source of pathogenic microorganisms. The use of disposable gowns, sheets, drapes, and pillow covers eliminates risks associated with cleaning and reuse of linens. Used linen, whether disposable or nondisposable, should be handled as little as possible and with minimum movement to prevent contamination of the air and of persons handling the linen, Figure 4-3.

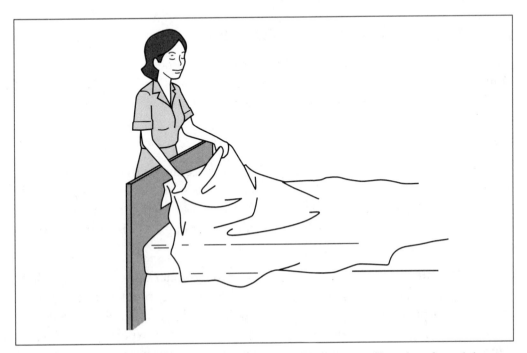

Figure 4-3   Handling linens. Linens should be unfolded, never flipped or fanned, because brisk movement stirs up air currents that carry microorganisms into the air.

All used linen should be bagged at the location where it is used. Do not sort or rinse linens in the patient care area. Linens soiled with blood or body fluids should be placed and transported in bags that prevent leakage.

Housekeeping. Housekeeping activities include cleaning environmental surfaces such as walls, floors, and other surfaces. Because these surfaces are not directly associated with the transmission of microorganisms to patients or others, attempts to disinfect or sterilize are not necessary; however, regular cleaning and soil removal must be performed.

Cleaning schedules and methods vary according to the type of medical facility, the particular service area, and the amount and type of soil present. Furniture and hard surfaced floors should be cleaned on a regular basis and when soiling or spills occur. Walls, window coverings, and blinds should be cleaned when they are visibly soiled. Vigorous cleaning and scrubbing with a disinfectant-detergent formula is considered effective against growth of microorganisms.

Disinfection

Disinfection is the destruction of microorganisms by using chemical methods. In radiography, disinfection methods are used on the radiographic table and certain equipment, accessories, and noninvasive articles. Commercially available disinfectant solutions may be used, but a solution of sodium hypochlorite (household bleach) is an inexpensive and effective germicide. Concentrations ranging from 1:100 dilution of household bleach to water are effective depending on the amount of organic material present on the surface. Regardless of the type or brand of disinfectant solution used, the following recommendations apply. (Information on specific label claims of commercial germicides can be obtained by writing to the Disinfectants Branch, Office of Pesticides, EPA, 401 M Street SW, Washington, DC 20460).

1. Read the directions provided for preparing and using disinfectants.
2. In patient-care areas, visible material should first be removed and then the area should be decontaminated. With large spills of cultured or concentrated infectious agents, the contaminated area should be flooded with a liquid germicide before cleaning, then decontaminated with a fresh germicidal chemical. Gloves should be worn during all cleaning and decontaminating procedures.

Common radiography items that require disinfection are the radiography table top as well as calipers, cassette surfaces, and immobilization aids.

Surgical Asepsis

Surgical asepsis includes procedures and techniques used to destroy micro-organisms before they enter the body. Such aseptic techniques are used whenever a surgical incision is made in the body. They are also used with invasive procedures, such as urinary catheterization, and when sterile instruments are handled and dressings are changed.

Surgical asepsis means that everything coming in contact with the patient is sterile. If an article is touched by an unsterile item, or if there is any question about the sterility of an item, it must be considered contaminated. Surgical asepsis is not generally used in procedures related to limited radiography procedures. For further information on surgical asepsis procedures, consult available nursing, health, and health assistant textbooks, which generally include donning sterile gloves, gowning, and preparing a sterile field.

RECOMMENDATIONS FOR THE PREVENTION OF THE SPREAD OF HUMAN IMMUNODEFICIENCY VIRUS (HIV)

AIDS and hepatitis B are just two of the many diseases that health care providers encounter in their daily work. The following suggestions include effective infection control measures for most other pathogens as well as HIV and hepatitis B. The suggestions are taken from the "Recommendations for Prevention of HIV Transmission in Health-Care Settings," published in the U.S. Department of Health and Human Services Centers for Disease Control publication, *Morbidity and Mortality Weekly Report,*[1] and "Update: Universal Precautions for Prevention of Transmission of Human Immunodeficiency Virus, Hepatitis B Virus, and Other Bloodborne Pathogens in Health-Care Settings."[2]

"Human immunodeficiency virus (HIV), the virus that causes acquired immunodeficiency syndrome (AIDS), is transmitted through sexual contact and exposure to infected blood or blood components and perinatally from mother to neonate. HIV has been isolated from blood, semen, vaginal secretions, saliva, tears, breast milk, cerebrospinal fluid, amniotic fluid, and urine and is likely to be isolated from other body fluids, secretions, and excretions. However, epidemiologic evidence has implicated only blood, semen, vaginal secretions, and possibly breast milk in transmission."

"The increasing prevalence of HIV increases the risk that health-care workers will be exposed to blood from patients infected with HIV, especially when blood and body-fluid precautions are not followed for all patients. *Thus health-care workers should consider all patients as potentially infected with HIV and/or other blood-borne pathogens and to adhere rigorously to infection-control precautions for minimizing the risk of exposure to blood and body fluids of all patients.*"

"*Universal Blood and Body Fluid Precautions*

1. All health-care workers should routinely use appropriate barrier precautions to prevent skin and mucus-membrane exposure when contact with blood or other body fluids of any patient is anticipated. Gloves should be worn for touching blood and body fluids, mucus membranes, or non-intact skin of all patients, for handling items or surfaces soiled with blood or body fluids, and for performing venipuncture. Gloves should be changed after contact with each patient. Masks and protective eyewear or face shields should be worn during procedures that are likely to generate droplets of blood or other body fluids to prevent exposure of mucous membranes of the mouth, nose, and eyes. Gowns or aprons should be worn during procedures that are likely to generate splashes of blood or other body fluids.

2. Hands and other skin surfaces should be washed immediately and thoroughly if contaminated with blood or other body fluids. Hands should be washed immediately after gloves are removed.

3. All health-care workers should take precautions to prevent injuries caused by needles, scalpels, and other sharp instruments or devices during procedures; when cleaning used instruments; during disposal of used needles; and when handling sharp instruments after procedures. To prevent needle-stick injuries, needles should not be recapped, purposely bent or broken by hand, removed from disposable syringes, or otherwise manipulated by hand. After they are used, disposable syringes and needles, scalpel blades, and other sharp items should be placed in puncture-resistant containers for disposal; the puncture-resistant containers should be located as close to the use area as practical. Large-bore reusable needles should be placed in a puncture-resistant container for transport to the reprocessing area.

4. Although saliva has not been implicated in HIV transmission, to minimize the need for emergency mouth-to-mouth resuscitation, mouthpieces, masks, resuscitation bags, or other ventilation devices should be available for use in areas in which the need for resuscitation is predictable.

5. Health-care workers who have exudative lesions or weeping dermatitis should refrain from all direct patient care and from handling patient-care equipment until the condition resolves.

6. Pregnant health-care workers are not known to be at greater risk of contracting HIV infection than health-care workers who are not pregnant; however, if a health-care worker develops HIV infection during pregnancy, the infant is at risk of infection resulting from perinatal transmission. Because of this risk, pregnant health-care workers should be especially familiar with and strictly adhere to precautions to minimize the risk of HIV transmission."

Implementation of universal blood and body-fluid precautions for *all* patients eliminates the need for use of the isolation category of "Blood and Body Fluid Precautions" previously recommended by the Centers for Disease Control and Prevention (CDC) for patients known or suspected to be infected with blood-borne pathogens.

Implementation of Recommended Precautions

Employers of health-care workers should ensure that policies exist for:

1. Initial orientation and continuing education and training of all health-care workers—including students and trainees—on the epidemiology, modes of transmission, and prevention of HIV and other blood-borne infections and the need for routine use of universal blood and body-fluid precautions for *all* patients.

2. Provision of equipment and supplies necessary to minimize the risk of infection with HIV and other blood-borne pathogens (gloves, gowns, masks, etc.).

3. Monitoring adherence to recommended protective measures. When monitoring reveals a failure to follow recommended precautions, counseling, education, and/or retraining should be provided, and, if necessary, appropriate disciplinary action should be considered.

Professional associations and labor organizations, through continuing education efforts, should emphasize the need for health-care workers to follow recommended precautions.

SAFETY MEASURES

Safety is the responsibility of everyone and must be an integral part of health care services. This concern includes not only the patient, but extends to everyone entering the health care facility. Accidents involving patients and staff can be reduced if simple safety measures are followed.

Preventing Falls

Patients may misjudge the distance from the radiographic examination table to the floor and fall as they attempt to get on and/or off the table. To reduce the likelihood of patient falls, you should always be at the table and provide a foot stool. Provide assistance also when the patient is getting on and off the table.

Tripping and falling account for numerous accidents. Protruding objects, loose scatter rugs, electrical cords, etc., should be removed or secured to prevent injuries. **Refer to Task 4-2 in the Appendix, Assisting the Falling Patient**.

Fire Safety

Fire safety begins with a fire safety plan that includes learning the location of fire doors, escape routes, and fire extinguishers, and knowing the evacuation procedure to follow during drills or the real thing. For further information, ask your supervisor about the facility's fire safety plan and participate in fire safety classes and evacuation drills.

Effective fire safety measures also include:

1. Smoking only in designated smoking areas
2. Fire inspections that try to uncover potential fire hazards before they cause fires
3. Annual preventative maintenance inspections on the heating and cooling units and other major electrical appliances/equipment
4. Installing smoke detectors and posting fire evacuation routes and fire exit signs
5. Regular checks on smoke detectors and fire extinguishers
6. Health-care workers who are constantly alert to potential fire hazards

Electrical Safety

Electrical safety involves proper use of electrical equipment and basic maintenance of the cords and circuits. Electrical equipment should be located away from sinks and other water reservoirs to avoid the possibility of electric shock. Electrical cords should be routinely inspected and broken or frayed cords replaced. Extension cords are a potential hazard and should not be overloaded with multiple appliances connected. Electric cords should not be draped around other items. A three-prong or safety plug provides added electrical grounding and is generally provided with heavy duty equipment or equipment that is in constant use, such as the electrocardiograph and laboratory centrifuge machines.

Accidents

Accidents do not just happen, they result from someone's inattention to details. Common sources of accidents are:

- Loose area rugs or torn carpet
- Unstable furniture or broken furniture
- Dangling electrical cords
- Young children or confused/disoriented person left alone/unattended
- Wet floors or highly waxed floors

The key to avoiding accidents is prevention. Each health worker should carefully look at his/ her work environment and reduce or eliminate potential accident conditions.

Reporting Accidents.   Accidents should be reported immediately to the staff supervisor. Each medical facility will have a procedure for reporting and recording accidents. Remember prevention is better than a cure. **Refer to Task 4-3 in the Appendix, Preparing Safety Reports (Accident/Incident).**

PRINCIPLES OF BODY MECHANICS

Health workers use physical effort to perform their jobs. Injury and fatigue are less likely to occur if proper body mechanics are used. Also, by applying the principles of body mechanics, limited radiographers can prevent patient injuries resulting from improper lifting and moving.

The term "body mechanics" refers to good posture, alignment of the body segments, and correct use of muscles or muscle groups. Good posture occurs when all parts of the body are in balance and each segment aligned, Figure 4-4. Good posture provides a balanced body that is steady and secure and less prone to improper muscle use, falls, and mishaps. In addition to a balanced stable body, good posture allows the internal organs to work with greater efficiency. The following are tips for good posture:

1. Stand with feet parallel and four to eight inches apart.
2. Keep body weight equally distributed on both feet.
3. Hold head erect with chin held in.
4. Hold chest and shoulders up.
5. Keep knees slightly bent.

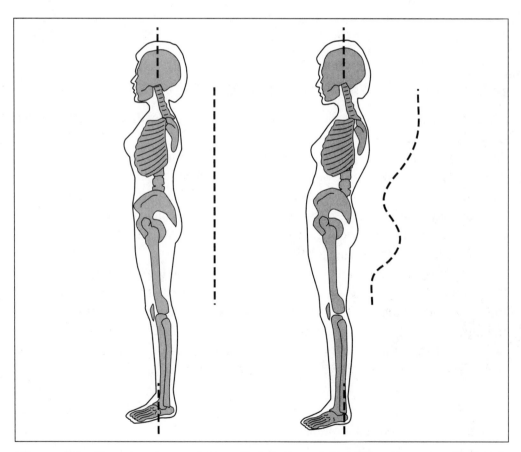

Figure 4-4 Correct posture, upright position. In the upright position, the center of gravity is the center of the pelvis

Good posture needs to be maintained during the performance of workday activities. Basic tips for good body mechanics during task performance are:

- Keep the body's line close to the center of gravity (the waistline) when moving or lifting patients or objects.
- Bend the knees when picking up an object from the floor. Do not bend from the waist.
- Pull weight with the upper arms using the biceps.
- Balance the load over both feet when lifting. Bring the patient or object close to the body, bend the knees, and set the spine to support the load. Use arm muscles to lift. Always keep body balanced. Do not twist the body to move with a load, rather change foot positions.
- Keep body balanced over feet and spread feet apart to provide a base of support.

MOVING AND TRANSPORTING PATIENTS

Limited radiographers work in a variety of settings and will encounter all kinds of patients. Examples of patient types follow.

Ambulatory patients—those who can walk and move. Ambulatory patients may require aides such as a walker, cane, or crutches.

Nonambulatory patients—those who cannot walk and move. Nonambulatory patients may arrive at the health care facility in an ambulance and be transported on a stretcher or a wheelchair. Ambulatory patients whose condition warrants may require transfer by wheelchair.

Before moving and transporting a patient, the radiographer must evaluate the patient's ability to aid in the process. Every patient must be considered in this evaluation since a patient's condition can change quickly. Generally, limited radiographers move and transport patients between a reception area or examination room to the radiography room and on and off the radiographic table. The following should be considered when assessing the patient:

- *General condition.* How does the patient appear? Is the patient alert, responsive, oriented, and functioning?
- *Mobility.* Did the patient walk into the facility without assistance? Are the patient's motions restricted in any way?

- *Strength and endurance.* Can the patient stand and walk without assistance? If so, will the patient become fatigued and be unable to complete the transfer without resting or assistance?
- *Balance.* Can the patient maintain balance? If the radiography procedure requires prolonged sitting or standing can the patient maintain the position without assistance?
- *Understanding and acceptance.* Does the patient understand the need to move and be transported? Does the patient seem willing and accepting of the move and transfer, or is the patient fearful?

After the initial assessment, the limited radiographer must decide what is the best way to move the patient and how much help will be required to safely make the move and transport. Never attempt to move or transport a patient without adequate assistance; to do so may cause injury to self or patient. It is helpful to remember the following rules related to patient transport:

- Move and transfer a patient over the shortest distance.
- Inform the patient about the move and ask for cooperation and help.
- Give short, simple commands.
- Give only the help the patient needs for safety and comfort.
- For standing and walking transfers, the patient should wear shoes.
- Lock all wheels on stretchers and wheelchairs before assisting the patient to move.

Trauma Radiography Guidelines

Patients who have experienced trauma may be unable to move and assume a position normally used for routine radiographic examinations. After the patient has been medically evaluated, it is the responsibility of the radiographer performing the examination to move the radiographic and accessory equipment around the patient so it will not cause the patient additional injury and discomfort. Each patient requires special attention and the following general trauma positions guidelines may be adapted to each situation.

1. Do not move the patient unless absolutely necessary
2. A minimum of two radiographs should be taken for each anatomic area. Try to obtain two radiographs at 90 degree angles to each other.

3. If the patient is conscious and coherent, explain exactly what is happening before beginning the radiographic examination.
4. Maintain the routine central ray entrance and exit point to as close to usual entrance and exit as possible.
5. Place the cassette adjacent to the part being radiographed to avoid magnification of the image.
6. Include both joints when possible on radiographs of long bones. If this is not possible, include the joint closest to the injury.
7. Do not remove splints or bandages unless instructed to do so.
8. Maintain intravenous fluid bottles above the level of the needle site.
9. Remove clothing from the unaffected side first.

Methods of Transfer

Patient transfer can be divided into ambulatory and nonambulatory methods and the skills and safety precautions associated with each.

Although a patient is ambulatory, an initial assessment should be conducted. It is the limited radiographer's responsibility to remain alert and observant of any change in status of the ambulatory patient and give assistance as needed.

The ambulatory patient should be provided with a footstool when getting on and off the radiography table. Also, it is best to walk with the ambulatory patient instead of way ahead or behind, just in case assistance is required.

In transferring nonambulatory patients, the limited radiographer must take great care to prevent further injury and to protect the skin. These patients may be handicapped, paralyzed, seriously injured, and/or unconscious. The body, head, and neck will require support during the move. Common methods of transfer include using a three-carrier lift, sheet transfer, and logrolling the patient. **Refer to Task 4-4 in the Appendix for the procedure for using a three-carrier lift, to Task 4-5 for the procedure for transferring a patient using a sheet, and to Task 4-6 for the procedure for logrolling the patient.**

Patients may use a walking aid to support their body. Patients with walking aids will require the greatest assistance when moving through heavy doors, narrow hallways, and especially in small dressing areas and in getting on and off the radiographic table.

Canes are used to provide balance and support when there is a weakness on one side of the body. A walker provides more support than a cane because it has four points of support. Limited radiographers should be alert to potential falls and loss of balance in the patient with a cane or walker. Should such an incident occur, the limited radiographer should provide support to the patient's weak side until she/he has regained support and balance on the cane or walker.

Crutches are used when one lower extremity is injured or when both extremities need strength. Patients with crutches are always at risk of falling because they must rest the upper arm weight on the crutches. When assisting the patient with crutches on and off the radiographic table, it is best to seek assistance and have support on both sides of the patient. **Refer to Task 4-7 in the Appendix for the procedure for assisting the patient with an ambulatory aid: cane, walker, and crutches. Also refer to the following tasks in the Appendix:**

Task 4-8 Transporting the Patient in a Wheelchair

Task 4-9 Transferring the Patient between Radiographic Table and Wheelchair

PATIENT HISTORY AND ASSESSMENT

The patient history assists the radiographer in knowing the extent of the injury, disease process, and ability of the patient to cooperate. The patient history also assists in the medical interpretation of the radiographs.

Certain disease processes or conditions require more or less radiation than the same healthy anatomic area. Some examples requiring a decrease in X-ray exposure are emphysema, osteoporosis, atrophy, and demineralization. Those requiring an increase in X-ray exposure are ascites, acromegaly, lung abscess, Paget's disease, pleural effusion, pneumonia, and an increase in bone mineralization.

Assessment of the patient means communicating with the patient about the procedure. Gaining the patient's confidence and trust though verbal and non-verbal communication is essential in the production of a high quality radiograph. From the moment a patient is greeted and their identification is established, the radiographer begins to develop a rapport with the patient but also begins to assess the patient. Assessment of the patient includes determining how much the patient will be able to assist during the radiographic procedure and whether modification of the routine is needed.

Often a patient's condition may not allow him or her to assume or maintain the routine or usual position for a particular X-ray examination. In these cases, the radiographer may be required to modify the usual procedure to provide the information requested. This may require different projections or central ray entrance, etc., however, the limited radiographer may not supply additional, unrequested positions without a medical request. The radiographer may consult with the attending physician to determine if additional positions, projections or views are necessary.

THE PATIENT'S RECORD: A RESOURCE DOCUMENT

Health care agencies use many types of forms for recording information about a patient. All of the forms used for a patient are placed in a folder and make up the patient's record. Charting is the process of making entries on the patient's record.

The patient's records serve many purposes:

- Guide to planning patient care
- Source of shared information that promotes continuity of the patient's care
- Source of information to keep all health personnel informed about the patient's care and condition
- Permanent summary of the patient's health status
- Research statistics
- Legal document

Making Entries on Patient Records

Each medical facility has certain guidelines about making entries on a patient's record. Such guidelines include who is responsible for writing on each form, the type of charting notations made, and what forms become part of the patient's permanent record.

Limited radiographers use patient records and make entries related to radiography procedures and basic patient care. Since limited radiographers generally function as a multiskilled professional, there may be many opportunities to refer to a patient's record and to make entries. Some examples are:

- The limited radiographer escorts a patient to the examination room, asks for the chief complaint, measures and records the vital signs, and enters the measurements on the patient record.
- The limited radiographer receives an oral telephone report on a special radiography procedure performed by a referral agency. The report is recorded and becomes part of the patient's record.
- The limited radiographer checks the chart to confirm the doctor's oral request for a radiograph.

Table 4-1 gives suggestions for making entries on a patient's medical record.

TABLE 4-1 ▪ Making Entries on Patient Medical Record

SUGGESTION	EXPLANATION
Use a pen to make entries.	The patient's record is a legal document and entries made in pencil can be too easily erased.
Make legible entries.	Write or print so others may read the penmanship. Illegible entries are useless.
Enter month, day, year.	Entries not properly dated lose their value as a source of information exchange and as a legal document. Many medical facilities also enter the time of day and AM or PM.
Follow facility policy concerning what should be recorded.	It is not necessary to record everything; follow facility policy.
Be brief and concise.	▪ Omit *a*, *an*, and *the*. ▪ Omit writing patient name. ▪ Use only standard common medical abbreviations.
Avoid personal judgment statements such as "seems like" or "appears to be." Quote the patient whenever possible. Record any adverse reactions, incidents, or mishaps the patient has.	If adverse reactions or unusual incidents are not recorded, it can be assumed they were not present. If the procedure or treatment requests are not documented as being carried out, it can be assumed they were not.
Some facilities require that documentation be made when ordered tests and procedures are completed. Describe instructions that a patient receives about examination preparation or self-administered contrast media. Do not rely on memory—record promptly.	Errors and omissions are likely if you rely on memory only.

continues

TABLE 4-1 ▪ (Continued)

Draw a line through an area left blank when not filled with information. Do not use ditto marks. Do not erase. Draw a single line through the error, write "error" near. Sign or initial all entries. Do not record for another person.	The line indicates that the area left blank was not intentionally omitted. Also, erasures may suggest falsification of information or facts.

MEETING PATIENTS' NEEDS

During any given day, a limited radiographer will provide care to a number of patients, each with a specific radiographic examination need. To complete the radiographs requested, patients may require assistance with meeting general and personal needs. Information related to meeting general and personal patient needs follows.

Physical Needs

Be aware of and provide for patients' privacy while they are dressing and undressing. Do not insist on staying with patients unless they ask for assistance or appear unable to help themselves. Knock on closed doors before entering, and close doors during procedures.

Limited radiographers may not notice how cool the room temperature feels because they are busy working; however, to the patient who may be disrobed, the room may be very cool. Provide a light blanket or sheet for the patient to use if he or she feels chilled.

Other Needs

Patient valuables, such as a purse, wallet, watch, jewelry, eyeglasses, dentures, prostheses, or other such items, should never be left unattended. Ask patients to keep these items with them at all times. If a patient's valuables are stolen, report this immediately to the supervisor.

Patients may need assistance in finding or ambulating to the bathroom. Bathrooms should be kept stocked at all times with adequate toilet paper, paper towels, soap, and sanitary pads. Patients who cannot ambulate to the bathroom, may require assistance or a urinal or a bedpan. Limited radiographers may require additional assistance in positioning a patient on a bedpan.

IV TUBES, URINARY CATHETERS, NASAL OXYGEN

Patients who have connecting IV tubes, urinary catheters, or nasal oxygen should be moved with care so as to not disturb these items. The limited radiographer's task is to take the required radiographs and to be observant of these items. If the IV tubing or urinary catheter becomes disconnected, it is important to report this immediately to the attending supervisor.

Limited radiographers often encounter patients who are receiving oxygen therapy. Without an adequate supply of oxygen in the body, metabolic activity decreases and life processes end. When individuals are unable to maintain a sufficient level of oxygen within their bodies, devices must be used to supplement their oxygen. It is safe to say that persons who require oxygen therapy are seriously ill and must be attended to carefully. An extremely important fact to remember is that *oxygen has properties that support combustion* and therefore becomes dangerous in the presence of sparks or flames. Although limited radiographers *do not* administer any type of oxygen therapy, it is important to recognize proper handling of patients receiving oxygen. Because oxygen is a highly combustible gas and radiographic equipment can cause sparks, the limited radiographer must always be extremely cautious and reduce the possibility of static electricity sparks when working where oxygen is being administered. Smoking is not allowed when oxygen is in use. Two common oxygen tanks are shown in Figure 4-5.

The amount of oxygen a patient is to receive is ordered by a physician. The various types of therapy devices are: (1) *nasal cannula* (Figure 4-6), (2) *nasal catheter*, (3) *face mask* (Figure 4-7), and (4) *oxygen tent*.

If an oxygen nasal cannula or face mask becomes dislodged or disconnected from the patient, the limited radiographer should put the nasal cannula or face mask back in place and ask the supervisor to check the equipment and the oxygen supply.

In most busy institutions where oxygen therapy is administered, experienced personnel are available to operate equipment and to provide assistance as needed.

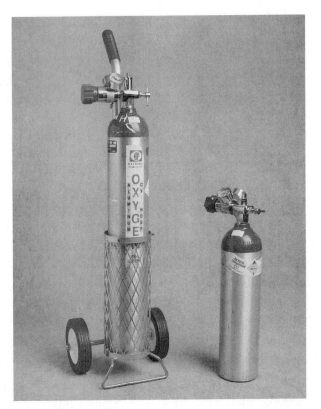

Figure 4-5   Oxygen tanks. Note gauge at top of tanks.

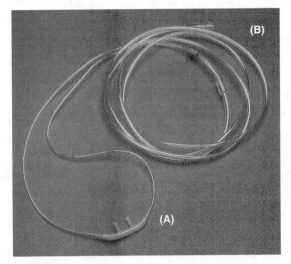

Figure 4-6   (A) Oxygen nasal cannula with (B) tubing.

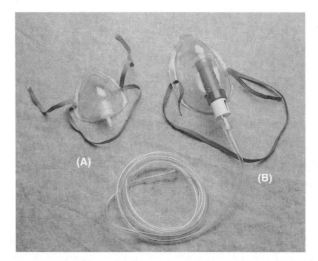

Figure 4-7 Oxygen masks (A) without tubing and (B) with tubing.

VITAL SIGNS

Limited radiographers must have knowledge of and be able to measure a patient's *vital signs*, i.e., those measures that let us know how a patient is doing on very basic levels of functioning—body temperature, pulse rate, blood pressure, and respiration rate. It is very important for limited radiographers to know the normal ranges of vital signs so that they can recognize deviations from the normal, which often indicate a medical emergency.

The definition of a medical emergency is a sudden, unexpected change in a person's vital functions that demands immediate action. In the medical setting, emergencies may not be unexpected if the patient has had appropriate clinical assessment and is receiving medical treatment. Accordingly, there may be signs that all medical personnel who come in contact with the patient should recognize—signs that indicate trouble or a change in the patient's condition. For example, a patient's lips turning blue is a sign of a serious loss of oxygen to the brain and requires immediate action. *Immediate action* is probably the most critical aspect of any emergency; it is the required spontaneous reaction to the situation that actually constitutes the emergency.

Vital signs are important and useful because they provide the first signs of trouble for a patient; they also gauge a patient's return to a stable condition following physiological disturbances.

Temperature

Body temperature is a reflection of heat production and loss. The normal or average body temperature of a healthy person is 98.6 F or 37 degrees centigrade. Average temperature may vary one to two degrees above or below 98.6 degrees F and still be within normal limits.

Body temperature is influenced by many factors. An increase in body temperature may be caused by a bacterial infection, physical activity, pregnancy, medication, and metabolism. A decrease in body temperature may be caused by a viral infection, exposure to cold and fasting.

A person is said to have a fever when their body temperature increases beyond their average or baseline temperature. The term *pyrexia* is synonymous for fever. Afebrile means without a fever. Fevers may be classified into four categories: (1) continuous, (2) remittent, (3) intermittent, or (4) relapsing. A continuous fever is one that does not fluctuate but remains above the person's average temperature for a period of time. A fever that fluctuates, rising above average and returning, is termed intermittent. A remittent fever never returns to average temperature but remains above average. A relapsing fever is one that returns after a period of being at the average or baseline temperature.

Four methods used for taking temperature are: (1) oral, (2) rectal, (3) axillary, and (4) aural. Temperatures may be measured by mercury or electronic thermometer, Figures 4-8 and 4-9, disposable thermometers, Figure 4-10, or a tympanic thermometer, Figure 4-11.

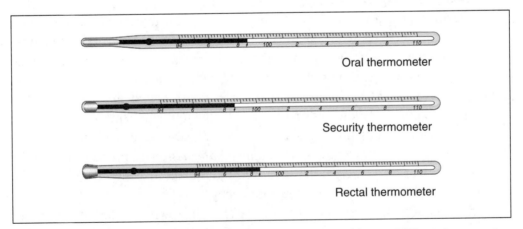

Figure 4-8 Clinical thermometers. *Top to bottom*: oral, security, rectal. These thermometers use the Fahrenheit scale of temperature measurement.

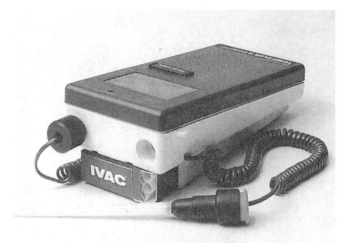

Figure 4-9 An electronic thermometer. The temperature is registered in large, easy-to-read numerals. The disposable protective sheath is placed over the probe tip. The probe is then placed in the patient's mouth in the usual manner. *(Courtesy IVAC Corporation)*

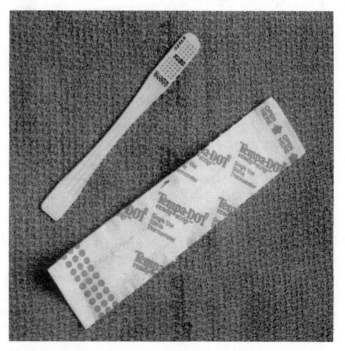

Figure 4-10 Disposable oral strip thermometer.

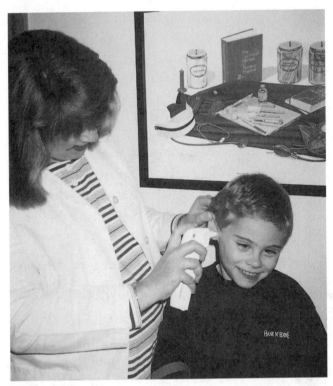

Figure 4-11 Measuring core body temperature with a
tympanic thermometer.

According to research findings from Children's National Medical Center in
Washington (1997), aural temperature is a more accurate and safer method for
checking children's temperature than all other methods.

To take a temperature orally, use an oral, glass tube, clinical thermometer with
an elongated tip. Before placing a thermometer in the patient's mouth, clean the
thermometer and shake the mercury down until it registers 96°F or below. The
thermometer should be placed under the tongue for three to five minutes with the
patient's mouth closed. If the patient has just ingested hot or cold liquids or foods
or has just smoked, wait fifteen to thirty minutes before taking the oral temperature. **Refer to Task 4-11 in the Appendix for the procedure for taking temperature using mercury, electronic, and tympanic thermometers.**

Use an oral thermometer to take axillary (under the arm) temperature. Leave the
thermometer in place for ten minutes in a dry armpit. This is the least reliable measure of temperature and generally is one degree lower than oral measurement.

To take temperature rectally, use a blunt tip (short, rounded) glass thermometer made specifically for rectal temperature measurement. This method is generally used on children or on adults whenever oral readings are uncertain. The thermometer is lubricated and placed within the rectum about one and one-half inches; it must be held in place two to three minutes. Red protective cover sheaths may be available to cover the thermometer. The temperature is generally one degree above oral measurement.

To provide an accurate temperature measurement using the tympanic thermometer proper positioning of the ear probe is critical. **Refer to Task 4-11 in the Appendix for the procedure for taking temperature using an aural thermometer.**

Pulse

Each beat of the heart is a pulsation that occurs when the heart contracts (tightens) to send blood through the arterial system. The beat or pulse may be felt at certain places on the body starting at the head and moving downward to the feet, Figure 4-12. The name and location of the different pulses are:

- *Temporal*—in front of the ear at the temple
- *Carotid*—in the front of the neck over the carotid artery
- *Apical*—actual heartbeat over apex of the heart; heard with a stethoscope
- *Brachial*—over the brachial artery at the inner surface of the elbow
- *Radial*—at the wrist just above the base of the thumb
- *Femoral*—in the groin over the femoral artery
- *Popliteal*—posterior or just behind the knee joint
- *Pedal*—on the arch of the foot at the dorsal pedal (dorsalis pedis) artery

The most common areas used to check pulse rate are (a) apical, with a stethoscope for accurate rate, and (b) radial, with the first two fingers placed on the inner side of the wrist at the depression just above the thumb. The farther away from the heart the pulse rate is taken, the more difficult it becomes to count because the pulse wave weakens.

Normal *pulse rates* range from fifty to one hundred beats per minute for adults. Many activities and events will cause a change in the heart rate, thus resulting in a change in the pulse rate. Table 4-2 shows average pulse beats per minute according to age groups. Pulse rates are affected by age, body build, exercise, medications (drugs), blood pressure, body temperature, pain, and various foods and liquids.

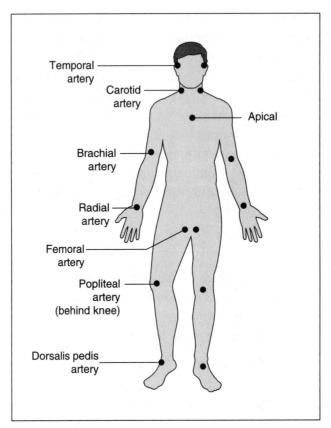

Figure 4-12   Pulse sites in the body.

TABLE 4-2 ▪ Average Pulse Beats per Minute According to Age Groups

	PULSE RATE PER MINUTE							
	Newborn	2 Years	4 Years	6 Years	8 Years	10 Years	12 Years	16 Years
Female	115–130	110	100	100	90	90	90	90
Male	115–130	110	100	100	90	90	85	75

There are several aspects to consider when checking pulse rates. A *regular* pulse has constant rhythm and equal time between pulses; this indicates good blood flow. An *irregular* pulse has inconsistent rhythm and may be felt as both strong and weak throbs. A *thready* pulse is weak, difficult to count, and irregular in rhythm; this pulse indicates poor blood flow. As stated earlier, when you are counting the radial pulse, place the tips of your first two fingers over the radial artery of the patient's wrist at the inner portion of the wrist just above the thumb and count the pulse beats for one minute. Do not apply your own thumb to the patient's wrist because the thumb has its own strong pulse. The procedure for pulse count is included with the procedure for counting respiration because pulse and respiration are generally checked together. **Refer to Task 4-12 in the Appendix for the procedure for counting the radial pulse and the respiratory rate.**

Respiration

The exchange of oxygen and carbon dioxide in the lungs is called respiration. Respiration occurs when a person takes in a breath (inhales) and lets out a breath (exhales). One such exchange is counted as one excursion of breathing. This exchange of gases is done at the rate of sixteen to twenty times a minute by the average adult.

Changes that occur in the chest during inhalation and exhalation are important considerations for the limited radiographer when doing a chest film. During chest radiography, it is important that the limited radiographer allow the patient to breathe in and out a couple of times to ensure that the lungs are fully inflated and that the diaphragm has moved down, allowing more lung to be visualized.

To reduce possible patient anxiety, it is best to count respirations when the patient is unaware that the count is being taken. The rate of breathing, like pulse, can be affected by such common considerations as age (children breathe faster, older people slower), exercise, emotions, disease, temperature, and medications.

Respirations may be counted after a patient's pulse has been taken. To do so, it is best to continue holding the wrist so the patient will not realize you are counting breathing excursions (inhalations and exhalations). To count respiration, count the number of times the patient's chest moves up or rises. Count respirations for sixty seconds. When observing a child, breathe with the child; this technique is particularly useful when you are making a radiographic exposure of the chest on full inhalation. It is equally important to listen to the patient's breathing to determine if it is labored or unusual in sound. Normal breathing should be relaxed, even and quiet. Respiration should be recorded as *regular*, *irregular*, *rapid*, *shallow*, or *labored*. Table 4-3 lists the medical term given to abnormal types of breathing and the characteristics of each.

Blood Pressure

Blood pressure (BP) is the force of the flow of blood exerted against the walls of the blood vessels. Blood pressure is measured by reading two numbers that register

---

TABLE 4-3 ▪ Abnormal Types of Breathing and Characteristics of Each Type

Apnea	Temporary cessation of breathing; suspended respiration.
Cheyne-Stokes	Bizarre breathing where apnea occurs from ten to sixty seconds followed by increased depth and frequency of breathing.
Dyspnea	Audible labored or difficult breathing.
Hyperventilation	Increased respiratory rate or breathing that is deeper than normal; forced respiration.
Orthopnea	Difficulty breathing while recumbent.
Otigopnea	A type of breathing that occurs in acute pulmonary disease when chest walls are thick; abnormally shallow or slow breathing.
Rales	Abnormal sounds heard in the chest, caused by air passage in the bronchi that contains secretion.
Spasmodic	Uneven
Stertorous	Labored
Stridor	Obstructed air passages that create a harsh sound during respiration; high-pitched sound like wind blowing.
Tachypnea	An increase in respiration rate; as in hyperventilation; abnormally rapid breathing.
Wheeze	Whistling sound as a result of narrowing of the lumen of respiratory passageway.

on an aneroid or mercury gauge called a sphygmomanometer, Figure 4-13.

Two numbers are read for blood pressure: (1) when the heart contracts or *systolic* pressure and (2) when the heart is relaxed or *diastolic* pressure. The average adult's blood pressure should be 120/80 mm of mercury. The top number (120) is the systolic pressure and the bottom number (80) is the diastolic pressure. Blood pressure is crucial to good health and may be affected by many things (Table 4-4).

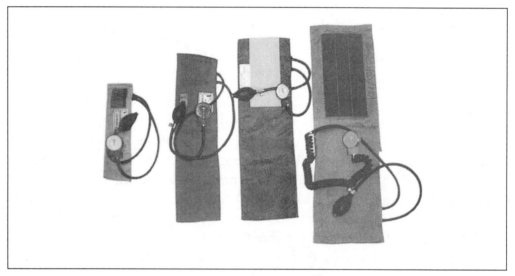

Figure 4-13 Aneroid manometer-type of sphygmomanometer for measuring blood pressure. Different size cuffs are shown. For an accurate measurement of blood pressure, it is important to use the proper size cuff on the patient. For example, a large adult cuff should not be used on a child.

TABLE 4-4 ▪ Average Blood Pressure According to Age Groups

		BP mm Hg						
	Newborn	2 Years	4 Years	6 Years	8 Years	10 Years	12 Years	16 Years
Female		98/60	98/60	98/64	104/68	110/72	114/74	120/78
Male		96/60	96/60	98/62	102/68	110/72	112/74	124/78

The same activities and events that affect the pulse also affect blood pressure. Other important situations prevalent in our society today that cause blood pressure problems are (1) heart and kidney disease, (2) vascular disease in the brain, (3) emotional conditions, (4) drugs, and (5) higher blood pressure in men than women in the same age group.

Hypertension and hypotension are two conditions with which the health professional needs to be familiar. *Hypertension* is high blood pressure created and exacerbated (made worse) by a variety of conditions including disease, emotional stress, and environmental stress. *Hypotension* is low blood pressure and is not necessarily an indication of illness unless the person has symptoms. However, low blood pressure related to shock or circulatory collapse is dangerous and can result in death if not treated.

To obtain an accurate blood pressure measurement, the limited radiographer must select the appropriate size cuff for the patient's arm. Cuff sizes range from newborn to obese and thigh cuffs are also available.

If the cuff size is too large the measurement will produce a false low reading. A cuff too small will produce a false high reading. The size of the blood pressure cuff should should be based on the patient's arm size and not on their age. Proper sizing for an adult cuff should allow for at least one-third to one-half the arm circumference. The length of the bladder should cover approximately 80% of the arm for adults and two-thirds of the upper arm of a child.

To ensure accurate readings, these rules must be followed:

1. Select the appropriate cuff size to fit the patient.
2. Inflate and deflate the cuff gradually.
3. Palpate the pulse before placing the stethoscope firmly over the brachial artery.
4. Ask the patient to be absolutely still.

Table 4-4 shows average blood pressures for age groups according to sex. Blood pressure will vary with age and physical condition. **Refer to Task 4-13 in the Appendix for the procedure for taking blood pressure.**

MEDICAL EMERGENCIES

Medical emergencies can and do occur in the office radiography environment. The limited radiographer must therefore have basic knowledge about medical emergencies and the immediate actions required.

Medical Emergencies Terminology

Shock: Shock is a failure of circulation in which blood pressure is inadequate to oxygenate tissues and remove by-products of metabolism. Symptoms of shock include restlessness, apprehension, fast pulse, pale skin, weakness, alteration in ability to think, cool, clammy skin, and systolic pressure below 30.

The radiographer's response to shock should be: Stop the procedure, place the patient in a recumbent (Trendelenburg position: head lower than the rest of the body), call for help, determine blood pressure, and administer oxygen if available. Do not leave the patient until help arrives.

Hypovolemic shock: Follows the loss of a large amount of blood or plasma.

Septic shock: Occurs when toxins produced during massive infection cause a dramatic drop in blood pressure.

Neurogenic shock: Causes blood to pool in peripheral vessels.

Cardiogenic shock: This is secondary to cardiac failure or other interferences with heart function.

Anaphylactic shock: A serious form of shock due to extreme sensitivity to a drug or foreign substance.

Anaphylactic reactions: May result in death. Patient may flush, exhibit hives, nausea, and loss of breathing.

Antigen: A protein that when introduced into the body causes formation of antibodies against it.

Epilepsy: A sudden passing disturbance of brain function.

Fainting: Temporary loss of consciousness due to loss of blood to the brain.

Hyperventilation: Increase in the amount of air entering the alveolar or air sacs.

Cardiac Tampondae: A collection of fluid or blood in the sac surrounding the heart which causes compression and prevents the heart from beating normally.

Cyanosis: A bluish discoloration.

Pulmonary Embolus: Obstruction of the pulmonary artery or one of its branches by undissolved matter.

Diaphoresis: Profuse perspiration

Eclampsia: Convulsion and coma occurring in a pregnant or newly delivered woman; rising blood pressure and protein in the urine are warning signals.

Uremia: The retention of excessive by-products of protein metabolism in the blood and the toxic condition produced by it.

DNR: Do Not Resuscitate

Syncope: (dizzy)

Stroke: **(CVA)** Cerebrovascular accident is an interference with blood supplied to the brain **(TIA)** a partial vessel occlusion and usually mild and temporary. **(Thrombus)** occurs when the cerebral vessel is totally occluded or ruptures, sudden loss of consciousness and one-sided paralysis (hemiparesis).

Vertigo: (sensation of having objects or the room spinning)

Fainting

Fainting is probably the most common emergency that occurs in the radiography setting. The limited radiographer must constantly observe all patients for signs of dizziness, pallor, or cold, clammy skin. At the first sign of fainting, have the patient lie down or place the head between the legs lower than the body. Application of cool compresses on the face may also be effective. Seek assistance as soon as possible.

Seizures

Seizures are caused by medical problems ranging from emotion or anxiety reactions to brain tumors. Epilepsy, usually found in children or young adults, is probably the most common cause of seizures. The most important response to a seizure is to make sure that the patient does not injure his/her head or body during the convulsive phase or obstruct his/her airway with his/her tongue. It is best to simply stay with the patient and call for assistance.

A mild seizure (petit mal) may be of short duration or may go unnoticed. A more severe seizure (grand mal) always requires assistance. Some symptoms of grand mal are jerky movements, rapid breathing, a loud cry, muscle rigidity, incontinence of urine or stool, vomiting, and frothing (foaming at the mouth). All symptoms that occur before, during, and after a seizure should be reported to a supervisor. The limited radiographer should make no attempt to open the patient's mouth or to force a solid object (such as wrapped tongue blades) into the mouth or airway.

Vomiting

Provide patient with a basin, tissue, and water for rinsing their mouth. If the patient is recumbent, turn the head to the side to prevent choking from aspiration of vomitus. If the patient is feeling nauseous, ask them to breath slowly and deeply through the mouth.

Nosebleeds (Epistaxis)

Bleeding or hemorrhage from the nose is usually referred to as epistaxis. *Universal Blood and Body Fluid Precautions* should be used when attempting to control bleeding. Nosebleeds may be controlled by applying external pressure to the side of the bleeding nostril. Cold compresses to the face may also be of value. The patient's head should be elevated. Seek assistance from the supervisor or attending physician.

Fractures and Spinal Injuries

Patients with these injuries should not be moved and supportive and restraining devices should not be removed. A physician must be present whenever the patient's position is changed.

Fractures.   A fracture is a break or rupture in a bone. Most fractures are the result of violent accidents or bone destruction caused by diseases. Fractures are classified by the type and extent of damage in the broken area. It is usually necessary to "reduce" a fracture, that is, to manipulate the broken ends so that the normal line of bone is restored. There are **two main classes of fractures: Open or compound and closed or simple**. An open fracture is one in which the broken bone protrudes through the skin, tearing the skin and soft tissues. A closed fracture is one in which the break in the bone is not accompanied by a break in the skin.

Fracture Terminology

Comminuted fracture: The bone has many fracture lines and is splintered into small fragments.

Transverse fracture: A straight break across the bone with only one fracture line.

Impaction: A type of fracture where one bone is driven into another portion of the same bone. The impacted fracture is common to the shoulder.

Pott's fracture: Common fracture to the distal tibia and fibula.

Greenstick fracture: The bone splits but does not break through completely, much the same as a piece of green wood.

Depressed fracture: A fracture in which the bone is driven inward, as in a skull fracture.

Pathological fracture: A fracture resulting from a weakening of the bone by chronic underlying disease which makes it more susceptible to breakage.

Avulsion fracture: The term *avulsion* means "to pull away from." Avulsion fractures generally occur at the point of a ligament or tendon attachment with a bone. The trauma results in a small piece of bone being pulled away from the main bone.

Colles' fracture: A fracture of the distal radius and a chip fracture of the ulnar styloid caused by trying to break one's fall by landing on an outstretched hand.

Intertrochanteric, transcervical, and subcapital fractures: Common fractures of the hip.

REVIEW QUESTIONS

1. Select the correct statements regarding nosocomial infections by placing a check mark (✔) beside the statement. A nosocomial infection
   _____ is generally acquired in hospitals or medical care settings
   _____ is more common in healthy adults
   _____ is considered opportunistic
   _____ can be reduced by using common asepsis

2. Asepsis is defined as the (circle the letter of the correct response)
   a) absence of all disease-producing organisms
   b) reduction of most disease-producing organisms

3. Match the following terms to the correct statement.
   _____ Surgical asepsis   a) reduction of microorganisms by using chemical methods
   _____ Disinfection   b) absence of all disease-producing organisms
   _____ Asepsis   c) procedures used to destroy microorganisms before they enter the body

4. Select the correct statement regarding the following. The Centers for Disease Control and Prevention recommends using universal precautions with (check one)
   _____ a) patients who appear ill
   _____ b) patients who have been diagnosed as HIV carriers
   _____ c) all patients regardless of their appearance or diagnosis

5. Normal adult body temperature when taken orally is (check one)
   _____ a) 96.6°F
   _____ b) 99.6°F
   _____ c) 97.6°F
   _____ d) 98.6°F

6. Normal adult pulse rate is within the range of (check one)
   _____ a) 50–70
   _____ b) 30–40
   _____ c) 80–100
   _____ d) 115–130

7. Normal adult blood pressure range is (check one)
   _____ a) 110/140
   _____ b) 126/150
   _____ c) 90/110
   _____ d) 70/80

8. Most people are free of infection most of the time because (check one)
   _____ a) there are few disease-causing organisms in the environment
   _____ b) microorganisms gain entrance to the body only through a break in the skin
   _____ c) microorganisms do not adhere to the skin of the body
   _____ d) the body's defense mechanisms protect it from invading germs

9. The limited radiographer should use the following body mechanics when lifting a patient
   1. keep the patient close to your body
   2. keep your back straight and do not twist at the trunk
   3. Stand with your feet together
      a) 1 only
      b) 1 and 2
      c) 1 and 3
      d) 1, 2, and 3

10. When cleaning the X-ray table, the limited radiographer should clean with
    a) a disinfectant after every use
    b) water and a dry cloth once a day
    c) antiseptic twice a day
    d) disinfectant once a week

11. Bleeding or hemorrhage from the nose is referred to as
    a) epistaxis
    b) hemostasis
    c) hemoplysis
    d) epiglossitis

12. To ensure accurate blood pressure readings, the limited radiographer should do all of the following, except:
    a) talk to the patient while taking the blood pressure reading
    b) select a cuff that fits the patient's arm
    c) palpate the pulse before placing the stethoscope over the artery
    d) Inflate and deflate the cuff gradually

13. Breathing where apnea occurs from ten to sixty seconds followed by increased depth and frequency of breathing is called
    a) apnea
    b) Cheyne-Stokes
    c) dyspnea
    d) stridor

14. A harsh high-pitched sound like wind blowing due to an obstructed airway is
    a) apnea
    b) Cheyne-Stokes
    c) dyspnea
    d) stridor

15. Difficult or labored breathing is called
    a) apnea
    b) Cheyne-Stokes
    c) dyspnea
    d) stridor

16. Temporary cessation of breathing is called
    a) apnea
    b) Cheyne-Stokes
    c) dyspnea
    d) stridor

17. Increased respiratory rate or breathing that is deeper than normal
    a) hyperventilation
    b) rales
    c) stridor
    d) wheeze

18. A pulse which is weak, difficult to count, and irregular in rhythm is called
    a) regular
    b) sycopated
    c) thready
    d) vascular

19. When taking a patient's pulse, the limited radiographer should observe all of the following, except
    a) apply the thumb and second finger to the patient's wrist
    b) recognize variations due to age, body build, exercise, medications
    c) count the pulse for one full minute and then record the reading
    d) pulse may be taken at the radial, femoral, popilteal or peadal areas.

20. All of the following are TRUE regarding a patient presenting with IV tubes, a urinary catheter, or nasal oxygen, except
    a) if an oxygen nasal cannula or face mask becomes dislodged from the patient, the radiographer should not attempt to put the nasal cannula or face mask back in place
    b) care must be taken to reduce the possibility of static electricity sparks and to prohibit smoking in areas where oxygen is being administered
    c) the radiographer should take precautions not to dislodge IV tubes, urinary catheters or nasal oxygen devices
    d) if IV tubing or a urinary catheter becomes disconnected, the radiographer should immediately report the situation to the attending supervisor.

21. Human immunodeficiency virus (HIV) has been scientifically proven to be transmitted through all of the following, except
    a) sexual contact
    b) semen and vaginal secretions
    c) breast milk
    d) shaking hands

22. What action should be taken by the limited radiographer if a patient's IV fluid runs out while the patient is receiving their radiographic procedure
    a) turn the IV off
    b) remove the IV from the patient
    c) call for the doctor or nurse
    d) no action is necessary

23. All of the following are correct regarding universal blood and body fluid precautions, except
    a) limited radiographers should routinely use barrier precautions to prevent skin and mucus-membrane exposure when contact with blood or other body fluids is anticipated
    b) never recap used needles, scalpels, or other sharps
    c) limited radiographers who have open lesions or weeping dermatitis should refrain from all direct patient care and equipment contact until the condition is resolved
    d) a limited radiographer may assume that a patient who tests negative for HIV is safe and can refrain from using universal blood and body fluid precautions with that patient.

For each type of shock, identify its causation factor or symptom.

24. ＿＿ anaphylaxis
25. ＿＿ cardiogenic
26. ＿＿ hypovolemic
27. ＿＿ septic
28. ＿＿ neurogenic

    a) occurs when a great amount of blood of plasma is lost
    b) blood pools in peripheral vessels
    c) a severe, life-threatening type of reaction to foreign proteins, i.e., bee sting
    d) caused by an infective condition resulting in extremely low blood pressure
    e) may occur with cardiac failure

29. The best thing to remember when attending to a patient who may have brain or spinal cord trauma is
    a) extreme pain may be caused if the patient is jolted
    b) brain and spinal cord injuries do not heal rapidly
    c) this type of trauma is susceptible to infections
    d) additional brain and spinal cord damage may be caused if the patient is moved.

30. If the patient displays signs and symptoms of vomiting while lying on the X-ray table
    a) have the patient roll over and lie face down
    b) assist the patient to turn their head to the side to avoid aspiration
    c) give the patient an emesis basin and escort them to the bathroom
    d) give the patient a drink of cola

31. A colle's type fracture would be most likely seen in a radiograph of the
    a) ankle   c) wrist
    b) knee   d) elbow

REFERENCES ━━━━━━━━━━━━━━━━━━━━━━━━━━━━━

1. *Morbidity and Mortality Weekly Report.* Centers for Disease Control. August 21, 1987, Vol. 36, No. 25. U.S. Department of Health and Human Services, Atlanta, GA.
2. "Update: Universal Precautions for Prevention of Transmission of Human Immunodeficiency Virus, Hepatitis B Virus, and Other Bloodborne Pathogens in Health-Care Settings," *Morbidity and Mortality Weekly Report*, Supplement. Centers for Disease Control. June 24, 1988, Vol. 37, No. 24, pp. 377–82, 387–88. U.S. Department of Health and Human Services, Atlanta, GA.
3. Torres, Lillian S., and Carol Morrill. *Basic Medical Techniques and Patient Care for Radiologic Technologists.* 2d ed. Philadelphia: J.B. Lippincott Company, 1983.

BIBLIOGRAPHY ━━━━━━━━━━━━━━━━━━━━━━━━━━━━

Answers About AIDS. A Report by the American Council on Science and Health. New York: American Council on Science and Health, 1988.

Atkinson, Lucy Jo and Nancymarie Howard Fortunato. *Operating Room Technique.* 8th ed. St. Louis: Mosby—Year Book, Inc., 1996

Cooper, Marian G., and David E. Cooper. *The Medical Assistant.* 5th ed. New York: McGraw-Hill Book Company, 1986.

Ehrlich, Ruth A., and Ellen M. Givens. *Patient Care in Radiology.* 2nd ed. St. Louis: The C. V. Mosby Company, 1985.

Fanning, Mary M.. *HIV Infection. A clinical Approach*, 2nd edition, Philadelphia, PA: W.B. Saunders Company, 1997.

Lindh, Wilburta Q., Marilyn S. Pooler, Carol D. Tamparo, Joanne U. Cerrato. *Comprehensive Medical Assisting: Administrative and Clinical Competencies.* Albany, NY: Delmar Publishers, 1998.

Miller, Benjamin F., and Clair B. Keane. *Encyclopedia and Dictionary of Medicine, Nursing, and Allied Health.* Philadelphia: W. B. Saunders Company, 1987.

Polaski, Arlene and Judith P. Warner. *Fundamentals for Nursing Assistants.* Philadelphia, PA: W. B. Saunders Company, 1994.

Rambo, Beverly J., and L. A. Wood. *Nursing Skills for Clinical Practice.* Philadelphia: W. B. Saunders Company, 1982.

Thomas, Clayton L. (Ed.). *Taber's Cyclopedic Medical Dictionary.* 15th ed. Philadelphia: F. A. Davis, 1985.

Chapter 5

Radiographic Physics

Chapter Outline

Objectives

Upon completion of the chapter, the student will meet the following objectives by verifying knowledge of the facts and principles presented through oral and written communication at a level deemed competent.

1. Identify the common units of measurement and atomic nomenclature.
2. Label an atomic illustration with the following energy shells: nucleus, proton, electron, neutron.
3. State the electric charge of a neutron, electron, and proton.
4. Draw an illustration showing atomic structure before and after ionization of the atom.
5. Identify the smallest unit of an atom, element, and compound.
6. List the origin and characteristics of electromagnetic radiation (gamma rays and X rays) and particulate radiation.

7. Identify the definition for the electrostatics and magnetism terminology list.

8. Match common electricity and magnetism laws and principles to their definition or application example.

"Why must I study physics?" and "How does physics relate to the everyday job of medical radiography?" are common questions asked by radiography students. Such questions express the students' need to understand how physics and related concepts apply to the everyday tasks performed by medical radiographers. One answer to these questions is that the basic laws and concepts of physics form the foundation of X-ray production, X-ray interaction, and radiographic image formation.

This chapter presents the essential laws and concepts of physics that have a direct application to medical radiography.

PART I: Natural Science Review

INTRODUCTION

Physics is a branch of science that deals with matter and energy and their relation to each other. It includes heat, sound, light, mechanics, electricity, magnetism, and the basic structure and properties of matter. Physics, like chemistry, astronomy, and geology, is considered one of the physical sciences and is classified as a natural science.

UNITS OF MEASUREMENT

Because physics is a science, it needs a way to accurately describe the physical reality with which it deals. This is accomplished with a system of measurement to describe physical quantities such as length, mass, or time. In the United States, the common measurement system uses units such as inches, feet, quarts, or pounds. The rest of the world, especially the scientific world, uses the International System of Units (SI units). These units are based on the familiar metric system where the meter is the standard of length, the kilogram is the standard of mass, and the second is the standard of time. All other SI units are derived from these few base units and are used to describe such quantities as area (square meters), velocity (meters/second), or volume (cubic meters). Other SI units based on more complex combinations of the base units are given special names such as the unit of force (the newton) or the unit of energy (the joule). The quantities of the units represented may be modified by the use of suitable prefixes. For example, a kilometer is 1000 meters and a millisecond is $\frac{1}{1000}$ of a second. Table 5-1 presents the base units, some of the derived units common to radiology and their special names, and the meaning of the prefixes used to modify the units.

TABLE 5-1 ▪ Systems of Measurement

British System	Foot, pound, second
Metric System	Centimeter, gram, second, meter, kilogram
SI System (International System of Units)	A new system of measurement in science that provides for the interconversion of units among all branches of science. Based on the metric system.
Units of Measurement	
Length	The unit of length. The *meter* (m) is the basic unit of length in the metric system.
Mass	A measurement of the quantity of matter in a body. The *kilogram* (kg) is the SI unit of mass.
Time	Measurement of intervals between events. The standard unit of time is *second*(s).
Area	Measurement of a given surface dependent upon length of area; square meters (m^2).
Volume	Measurement of the capacity of a container, dependent upon length of container. Volume may be expressed in cubic meters (m^3), liters (l), milliliters (ml), or cubic centimeters (cc or cm^3).
Velocity	Speed in a given direction. Expressed in meters per second (m/s).
Temperature	Expressed as degrees Celsius or Fahrenheit. Celsius = 0°C freezing point of water 100°C boiling point of water Fahrenheit = 32°F freezing point of water 212°F boiling point of water

CONCEPTS OF MATTER

The universe consists of matter and energy. Matter may be defined in terms of its properties such as mass or volume. **Energy** is the ability to do work, where work is defined as the application of force over a distance. There are many different forms of energy, such as mechanical, electrical, or heat. There are two types of the various forms of energy: kinetic and potential.

Kinetic energy is energy of motion. When an object is moving, it possesses kinetic energy. Examples of kinetic energy are a pitched baseball, a moving automobile, or a person walking. Because any moving object possesses two quantities, mass and velocity, kinetic energy is expressed in terms of mass and velocity.

Potential energy is stored energy. Potential energy exists because of an object's position. For this reason, it is called energy of position. On the earth, an object's potential energy depends on its height above the ground. Any object may possess either kinetic energy or potential energy or both. For example, if a person holds a ball above the ground, it will have potential energy by virtue of its height. However, it will have zero kinetic energy because it is not moving. If the ball is dropped and is falling, it will possess kinetic energy because of its motion and it will also have potential energy because it is still above the ground. At the instant the ball strikes the ground, the kinetic energy will be at its maximum while the potential energy will be zero.

The **Law of Conservation of Energy** states that energy can be neither created nor destroyed but can be changed into other forms of energy. Some different types of energy are mechanical, thermal, radiant, electrical, chemical, and nuclear, and change can occur between these forms. The change of energy from one form to another is called a transformation of energy. Figure 5-1 gives examples of energy transformation.

While energy can exist in many different forms, matter exists in only three states: solid, liquid, and gas. Matter can be converted from one state to another, depending upon conditions of pressure and temperature. For example, water is a liquid form of matter. However, when it is subjected to freezing temperatures, the state of water is converted into a solid—ice. Heated to boiling, water becomes a gas in the form of steam. Matter can be in either a state of rest (inertia) or motion (momentum). Matter is described by the physical quantities associated with these states, such as mass, volume, or temperature.

Three States of Matter

Solid	Liquid	Gas
Ice	Water	Steam

Energy Transformation

Baking powder/yeast	Causes baking mixtures to rise.
Chemical battery	Coverts to electrical energy to power a flashlight or radio.
Sunlight	Captured in photosensitive solar cells for conversion to electricity.

Figure 5-1   Examples of matter and energy transformation

All matter is composed of atoms. The **atom** is the smallest particle into which matter can be divided while still maintaining a unique identity. The identities of different types of matter are distinguished by how they react chemically. Atoms that have different chemistries are considered distinct **elements**. There are presently 109 separate elements. The atomic and chemical relationship of one element to another follows a regular pattern that is described by the **Periodic Table of Elements**, Figure 5-2. All elements in the same vertical column (group) will chemically respond in a similar manner.

Atoms of the same or different elements may be chemically combined to form **molecules**. Molecules, which themselves have distinct physical properties, form the basis for the complex chemical substances called **compounds**. For example, two atoms of hydrogen associate to form a molecule of hydrogen gas. When two atoms of hydrogen **associate**, or bond, with one atom of oxygen a molecule of water is formed, Figure 5-3. Many molecules of water form the compound water with which we are familiar and that may be described by such physical properties as its freezing point (0°C, 32°F) and boiling point (100°C, 212°F).

ATOMIC STRUCTURE

The atom, the basis for the elements, is itself made up of separate particles. All atoms are composed of three fundamental particles: the proton, the neutron, and

PERIODIC TABLE OF THE ELEMENTS

Legend:
- 6 — Atomic Number
- C — Element Symbol
- 12 — Atomic Mass Number

Group / Period	I	II											III	IV	V	VI	VII	VIII
1	1 H 1																	2 He 4
2	3 Li 7	4 Be 9											5 B 11	6 C 12	7 N 14	8 O 16	9 F 19	10 Ne 20
3	11 Na 23	12 Mg 24											13 Al 27	14 Si 28	15 P 31	16 S 32	17 Cl 36	18 A 40
4	19 K 39	20 Ca 40	21 Sc 45	22 Ti 48	23 V 51	24 Cr 52	25 Mn 55	26 Fe 56	27 Co 59	28 Ni 59	29 Cu 64	30 Zn 65	31 Ga 70	32 Ge 73	33 As 75	34 Se 79	35 Br 80	36 Kr 84
5	37 Rb 86	38 Sr 88	39 Y 89	40 Zr 91	41 Nb 93	42 Mo 96	43 Tc 99	44 Ru 101	45 Rh 103	46 Pd 106	47 Ag 108	48 Cd 112	49 In 115	50 Sn 119	51 Sb 122	52 Te 128	53 I 127	54 Xe 131
6	55 Cs 133	56 Ba 137	57 to 71	72 Hf 179	73 Ta 181	74 W 184	75 Re 186	76 Os 190	77 Ir 192	78 Pt 195	79 Au 197	80 Hg 201	81 Tl 204	82 Pb 207	83 Bi 209	84 Po 210	85 At 210	86 Rn 222
7	87 Fr 223	88 Ra 226	89 to 109															

Note: Elements 57 to 71 are the rare earth metals.

Elements 89 to 109 are the actinide metals.

Figure 5-2 Periodic Table of the Elements

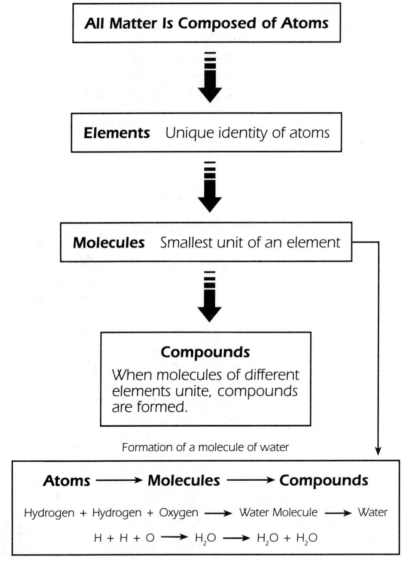

Figure 5-3   Matter composed of atoms and formation of a molecule of water

the electron. The **proton** and the **neutron** are found in the center of the atom, called the **nucleus**, and have approximately the same mass. The proton has one positive electrical charge and the neutron is uncharged. For each positively charged proton in the nucleus of an uncharged atom there is one negatively charged (and much less massive) **electron** outside the nucleus, Figure 5-4. Since the number of positive

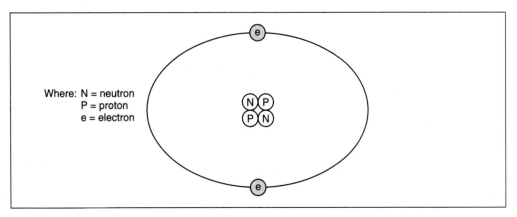

Figure 5-4   A simplified model of a helium atom

particles (protons) in an atom equals the number of negative particles (electrons), the atom as a whole exists in an uncharged, or neutral, state.

The number of protons in an atom is called the **atomic number** (abbreviated Z) and the number of protons plus neutrons is the **atomic mass number** (A). Atoms are arranged on the periodic table by order of increasing atomic numbers.

Electrons exist in discrete positions outside the nucleus. These positions are called **orbitals** and represent the amount of energy individual electrons possess. Just as atoms of individual elements are arranged in the periodic table according to their atomic structure, electrons are arranged in a systematic fashion around the nucleus of an atom. Electrons are bound to atoms by an amount of energy, called the **electron binding energy**, which varies according to the position of the electrons. Electrons closest to the nucleus have the most binding energy and those farthest away the least. The orbitals in which the electrons are bound represent different energy levels. Each energy level, or shell, is designated by a different letter of the alphabet, beginning with the K-shell, closest to the nucleus, and proceeding through the L-, M-, N-, O-, P-, and Q-shells outward from the nucleus, Figure 5-5.

The numbers of electrons that can occupy each shell also follow a set of rules. If each electron shell is given a number starting with one for the K-shell, two for the L-shell, and so on, the maximum number of electrons that can fill that shell is given by the formula

$$2n^2 \text{ (2n(squared))}$$

Where: n is the number of the electron shell. Therefore, only two electrons are allowed in the K-shell, eight in the L-shell, and up to ninety-eight in the Q-shell.

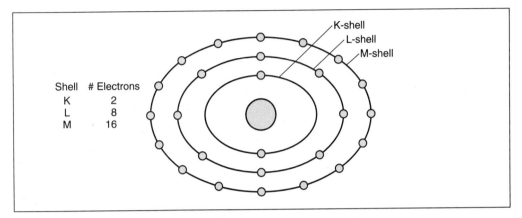

Figure 5-5 The electron shells of a sulfur atom

Another rule states that the maximum number of electrons allowed in the outer shell is eight.

The number of electrons in the outer shell is related to the position of an element on the periodic table, with the number of outer shell electrons increasing from left to right. As it is the outer-shell electrons that determine the chemical reactivity of an atom, elements that chemically respond in a similar manner are found in the same vertical column of the periodic table.

ATOMIC NOMEMCLATURE

Elements are commonly shown in an alphabetic abbreviation. This is the **chemical symbol** of the element as shown in Table 5-2. To further distinguish separate elements, the atomic number (the number of protons) is written as a subscript to the left of the chemical symbol and the atomic mass number is written as a superscript to the left of the chemical symbol, Figure 5-6.

Atoms of the same element may have different numbers of neutrons in the nucleus while maintaining the same chemical identity. Atoms that have the same number of protons but different numbers of neutrons are called **isotopes**. Hydrogen is the simplest element, with a nucleus of one proton and one orbital electron. A neutron can be added to the nucleus of hydrogen, thus giving an atomic mass number of two (one proton + one neutron). This atom is called deuterium, Figure 5-7. Chemically it is the same as hydrogen because it has one proton and one electron, but atomically it is different (an isotope of hydrogen) because it has one neutron.

TABLE 5-2 ▪ Elements Important to Radiology

CHEMICAL SYMBOL	ELEMENT	ATOMIC NUMBER (Z)	ATOMIC MASS NUMBER (A)
C	Carbon	6	12
O	Oxygen	8	16
Al	Aluminum	13	27
Ca	Calcium	20	40
Fe	Iron	26	56
Cu	Copper	29	63
Mo	Molybdenum	42	98
Ru	Ruthenium	44	102
Ag	Silver	47	107
Sn	Tin	50	120
I	Iodine	53	127
Ba	Barium	56	138
W	Tungsten	74	184
Pb	Lead	82	208

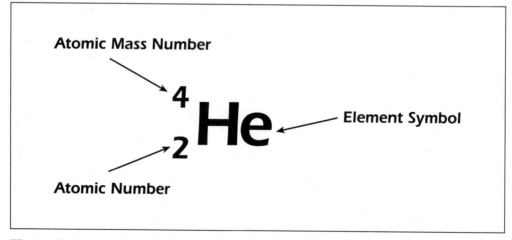

Figure 5-6 Atomic symbol nomenclature

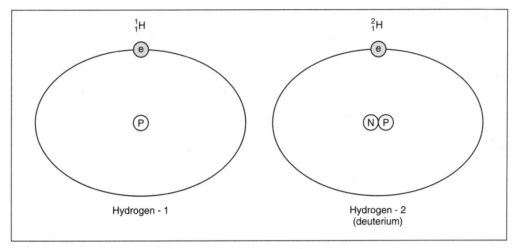

Figure 5-7   Two isotopes of hydrogen

IONIZATION

Atoms are electrically neutral, their electric charge being zero, because the total number of protons is equal to the number of electrons in the orbital shells. An atom may become **ionized** if it gains or loses an electron. Any charged particle is an **ion**. The loss of an electron results in a net positive charge and the atom is termed a **cation**. The addition of an electron to an atom results in a net negative charge and the atom is called an **anion**. An electron may be removed from an atom by the addition of energy to the atom. When this happens the removed electron and the electron from which it is removed are called an ion pair, Figure 5-8.

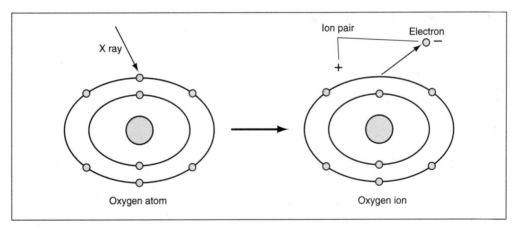

Figure 5-8   Ionization of an oxygen atom by an X ray

Types of Ionizing Radiation

Radiation is simply defined as the process of emitting radiant energy in the form of waves or particles. Radiation may be classified as either **ionizing** or **non-ionizing**. If radiation is in the form of matter, it is called **particulate radiation**. If the radiation is in the form of pure energy, that is without mass and charge, it is called **electromagnetic radiation**. Since either type of radiation is capable of ionizing atoms, this radiation is collectively called ionizing radiation. Table 5-3.

When ionizing radiation passes through matter, positively and negatively charged particles (ions) are produced and the ionization has occurred. Non-ionizing radiation does not cause the production of these charged particles. Examples of non-ionizing radiation are microwaves, radio waves, and ultraviolet rays.

TABLE 5-3 ▪ Ionizing Radiation

PARTICULATE

Subatomic particles in motion that originate from the nucleus of radioactive atoms. Radioactive atoms have nuclei that contain excess energy and particles. In an attempt to regain stability, these radioactive atoms emit their excess energy and particles.

RADIOACTIVE DECAY PROCESS

Alpha Particles	Beta Particles
(equivalent to two neutrons)	(equivalent to an electron)
can travel 5 cm	can travel 10–100 cm

Traveling particles of radiation

ELECTROMAGNETIC

Electromagnetic radiation differs from particulate in that it consists of bundles of energy (photons) and travels in wavelength form.

Two Types

Gamma radiation, like particulate radiation, originates from nucleus of radioactive atoms; however, it differs in that it exists as wavelengths of energy and is very penetrating to humans.

X ray is similar to gamma, but originates in orbitals.

Ionizing radiation may be from a natural source or artificial (man-made) source. Radioactive materials in the earth such as uranium, radium, and thorium, cosmic radiation, and radionuclides in the environment are sources of natural background radiation. X-radiation is a man-made source of radiation and is classified as ionizing radiation because of its ability to create electrically charged particles as it passes through matter. These electrically charged particles possess the potential to cause biological damage in living tissue, thus creating the need for radiation protection practices.

PARTICULATE AND ELECTROMAGNETIC RADIATION

Particulate radiation may occur as any of the common subatomic particles or as ionized atoms. Two common types of particulate radiation are alpha particles and beta particles. **Alpha particles**, or alpha rays, are the nuclei of helium atoms, two protons and two neutrons, and therefore have a charge of +2. **Beta particles** (beta rays) are physically identical to electrons. Both alpha particles and beta particles have the ability to remove electrons from atoms, thus ionizing the atoms.

The matter of the universe exists in a sea of energy. Much of this energy is in the form of electromagnetic radiation. There are many types of electromagnetic radiation, such as visible light, radiowaves, or X rays. Electromagnetic radiation has no mass and no charge. It exists in the form of waves and may be described as a wave, Figure 5-9. If one considers the wave form in Figure 5-9, the distance from the peak of one wave to the next is the **wavelength** and is measured in meters. The height of a wave from the lowest valley to the highest peak is the **amplitude**. The part of a wave followed from halfway between a peak and valley up through the next peak and down through the next valley to the next midpoint is called one **cycle**. The number of cycles passing through a given point in one second is the **frequency**. The frequency is measured in cycles/second, given the name Hertz in SI units, and abbreviated Hz.

Electromagnetic radiation is described by the three quantities of wavelength, frequency, and energy. The entire energy-frequency-wavelength range of electromagnetic radiation is known as the **electromagnetic spectrum**, Figure 5-10.

As may be seen from Figure 5-10, there are many different types of electromagnetic radiation. Visible light, to which the human eye responds, is intermediate on the electromagnetic spectrum in energy. Just below visible light are infrared radiation, which some insects can see; microwaves, used in cooking and

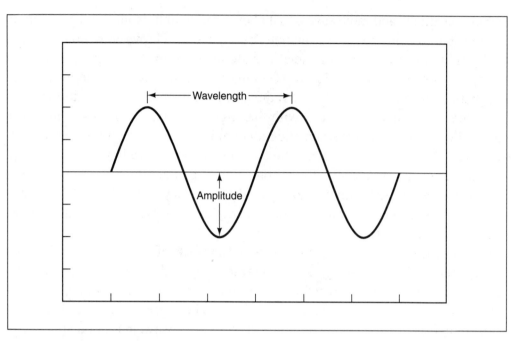

Figure 5-9 Amplitude and wavelength

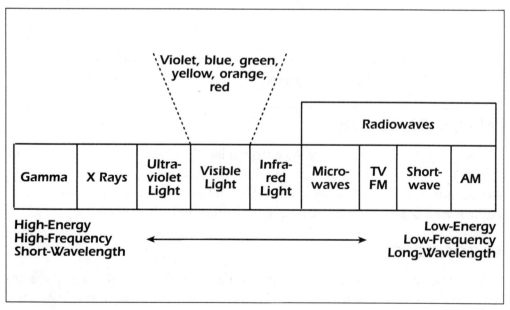

Figure 5-10 The electromagnetic spectrum

communications; and radiowaves. Just above visible light is ultraviolet radiation, responsible to some extent for human "sun-tanning." Above ultraviolet, X rays and gamma rays are found. Gamma rays are identical to X rays in every respect except in how they are produced. (Gamma radiation is a high-energy electromagnetic radiation resulting from a radioactive decay process. X-radiation results from the interaction of electrons with the target material of an X-ray tube.) The higher the energy of electromagnetic radiation is, the better it can penetrate matter. Thus, X rays are used to penetrate the human body for radiographic imaging.

The energy and frequency of electromagnetic radiation are directly related— that is, the higher the energy is, the higher the frequency is. Energy and frequency are inversely related to wavelength: the higher the energy or frequency is, the shorter the wavelength.

Electromagnetic radiation is not one continuous waveform but instead consists of separate packets of energy called **quanta** (singular quantum) or more commonly **photons**. A photon may be thought of as a massless, uncharged bundle of energy that has properties of continuous waves. Therefore, X rays are commonly spoken of as photons or X-ray photons. Photons are always in motion and always travel at the same velocity in a vacuum—300 million meters/second (186,000 miles/second). Since visible light is a type of electromagnetic radiation, this velocity is called the **speed of light**.

PART II: Electricity and Magnetism

INTRODUCTION

Electricity is a form of energy. As energy it has the ability to do work. The work electricity does in an X-ray machine is the production of electromagnetic radiation in the form of X rays. To understand how this occurs, one must first know something of the basic nature of electricity and magnetism.

ELECTRICITY

All atoms and subatomic particles have either a presence or absence of electrical charge. Protons have a single positive charge, electrons have a single negative charge, and neutrons have no charge. Atoms may have no charge, be singly charged, or have more than one charge, as long as the charge is a whole number (integer). Electrical charges obey certain physical laws, the most important being that like charges repel each other and unlike charges attract each other. A proton will be repelled by another proton but will attract an electron.

When an object has an electrical charge, it is said to be electrified or statically charged. The phenomenon of charged objects is termed **electrostatics** or **static electricity**. Electrification results from either a deficiency or an excess of electrons and occurs when electrons move from one object to another, Figure 5-11. The amount of electrification is measured in a unit called the **coulomb (C)**, which represents 6.3×10^{18} electron charges. Positive charges do not move except in special cases involving ionized atoms.

The study of moving electrical charges is called **electrodynamics**. The movement of electrical charges, or electrons, occurs from one atom to another along the outside of a conductor. A **conductor** is a material that allows the easy movement of electrons. Most metals, such as copper, are good conductors. Materials, such as rubber or plastic, which impede the flow of electrons, are called **insulators**, Figure 5-12.

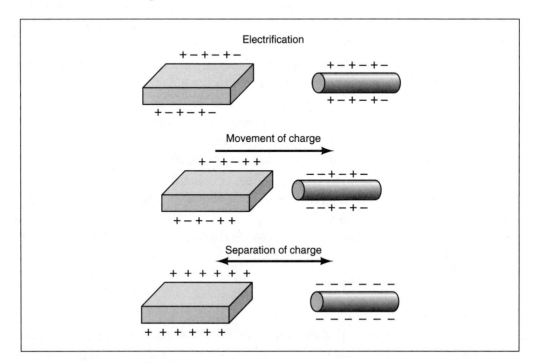

Figure 5-11   Electrification

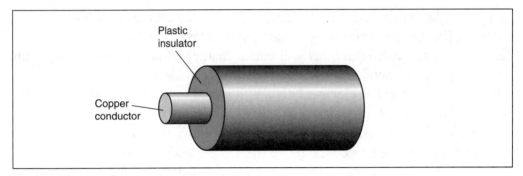

Figure 5-12 Typical electrical wire

Electrical charges possess potential energy because they have the ability to do work by virtue of the repulsion of like charges and the attraction of unlike charges. This potential of electrical charges to do work is called **electrical potential**. The difference in electrical potential between two points on an electrical conductor is called the **potential difference**. This is analogous to mechanical potential energy. An object positioned above the ground has more potential energy than the same object on the ground because of the difference in height, or gravitational energy. In the same fashion, electrons at one end of a conductor have the ability to do work because they are repelling each other.

If a conductor is connected to a source of electrons, such as one end of a battery, and is connected to the other end of the battery to form an electrical circuit, electrons will flow along the conductor and work will be done. The amount of work performed by moving electrical charges is measured in volts (V). Electrons moving through a conductor are called **current**, which is measured in amperes (A).

If a circuit is modified to resist the flow of electrons, work can be extracted from the circuit in various forms, such as heat or radiant energy. Electrical resistance is measured in ohms (Ω). An **ohm** is the amount of resistance overcome by one volt to cause one ampere to flow.

The product of current (amperes) and resistance (ohms) is volts. This equation is expressed as:

$$V = IR$$

Where: V = voltage in volts, I = current in amperes, and R = resistance in ohms. This is called **Ohm's law** and forms the basis for the study of electrical circuits.

The amount of work that electricity does over a given amount of time is called **power** and is measured in watts (W).

MAGNETISM

Magnetism is the ability of some material to attract iron or ironlike substances. The magnetic property of a substance is defined by the magnetic field it creates. The magnetic field is the zone of influence of the magnetic property and is concentrated at two points called the **magnetic poles**. The earth itself is a huge magnet which has its magnetic poles at the geographical north and south. In a similar fashion, the poles of all magnets are called the north and south poles. A basic law of magnetism states that like poles repel each other and unlike poles attract each other.

Magnets may be naturally occurring substances or may be created by passing an electrical current through a conductor. This type of electromagnet is important in the operation of X-radiation generating equipment and will be discussed further in Chapter 7.

REVIEW QUESTIONS ━━━━━━━━━━━━━━━━━━

1. In ionization
   a) an electron may be removed from an atom
   b) a proton may be removed from an atom
   c) a neutron may be removed from an atom
   d) two of the above
2. Which of the following is a particulate radiation?
   a) X ray
   b) beta ray
   c) gamma ray
   d) two of the above
3. Which of the following statements is FALSE?
   a) A neutron has no charge.
   b) A proton has a positive charge.
   c) A neutron has approximately the same mass as an electron.
   d) A neutron has approximately the same mass as a proton.
4. Compounds are composed of _____ and molecules are composed of _____.
   a) atoms, molecules
   b) molecules, neutrons
   c) molecules, atoms
   d) nucleons, atoms

5. How many atoms are there in one molecule of H_2O?
   a) 1
   b) 2
   c) 3
   d) 4

6. The SI unit of mass is the
   a) gram
   b) kilogram
   c) meter
   d) pound

7. Compared to radiowaves, X rays and gamma rays have
   1. higher energy and longer wavelength
   2. higher energy and shorter wavelength
   3. higher frequency and shorter wavelength
      a) 1 and 2
      b) 1 and 3
      c) 2 and 3
      d) 1, 2, and 3

8. Electrification occurs because of
   a) the movement of protons
   b) the movement of neutrons
   c) the movement of electrons
   d) the movement of atoms

9. Electric charge is measured in
   a) amperes
   b) coulombs
   c) volts
   d) ohms

10. Amperage is a measure of
    a) current
    b) force
    c) resistance
    d) charge

11. All of the following are TRUE, except
    a) radiation having matter and form is called particulate
    b) radiation is pure energy
    c) ionized atoms cause particulate radiation
    d) alpha and beta are examples of electromagnetic radiation
12. All of the following relate to the Law of Conservation of Energy, except
    a) energy may be changed into other forms of energy but neither created nor destroyed
    b) when energy is changed from one form to another it is said to be transformed
    c) matter can be either in a state of inertia or momentum
    d) is another form of the periodic table of elements
13. If radiation exists in the form of matter, it is referred to as
    a) super charged
    b) electromagnetic
    c) particulate
    d) cantionized
14. If radiation exists in the form of pure energy, it is referred to as
    a) super charged
    b) electromagnetic
    c) particulate
    d) cantionized

BIBLIOGRAPHY

Bushong, Stewart C. *Radiologic Science for Technologists Physics, Biology, and Protection*, 6th ed. St. Louis: The C. V. Mosby Company, 1997.

Carlton, Richard R. and Arlene M. Adler. *Principles of Radiographic Imaging, An Art and a Science*, 2nd ed. Albany, NY: Delmar Publishers, 1996.

Currey, Thomas S., James E. Dowdey, and Robert C. Murry. *Christensen's Physics of Diagnostic Radiologic*. Philadelphia: Lea & Febiger, 1990.

Pizzutiello, Robert and John E. Cullinan for Eastman Kodak. *Introduction to Medical Radiographic Imaging*. Rochester, NY: Eastman Kodak Company, 1993.

Selman, Joseph. *The Fundamentals of X-Ray and Radium Physics*, 7th ed. Springfield, Illinois: Charles C. Thomas, Publisher, 1985.

Chapter 6

Radiographic Tube and Radiation Production

Chapter Outline

Introduction
Radiographic-Tube Construction
The Line Focus Principle
Tube Rating Charts
Tube Heat Capacity

Objectives

Upon completion of the chapter, the student will meet the following objectives by verifying knowledge of the facts and principles presented through oral and written communication at a level deemed competent.

1. Describe and explain the function of the components of the radiographic tube as they relate to radiation production.
2. Describe radiographic tube heat production and show how to calculate its related heat capacity.
3. Explain the process by which radiation is produced from the conduction of electrons within the tube.
4. Explain radiographic tube stability related to heat production.

INTRODUCTION

In radiography, the X-ray machine is the primary instrument, and the radiographic tube is the most important part of this instrument. Yet, in day-to-day work, the radiographic tube is too often taken for granted—we tend to think the tube always functions properly until one day it no longer functions at all and has to be replaced. Generally, the tube seems to withstand a great deal of usage (and at times, abuse) but a knowledge of its operation can prevent many of the causes of tube failure.

RADIOGRAPHIC-TUBE CONSTRUCTION

The **X-ray tube** is a relatively simple instrument. Its structure consists of an outer metal housing, which serves as protection for the glass tube inserted within that housing, Figure 6-1. On one side of the tube is a source of electrons, the **cathode**. On the other side of the tube is the target for the electrons, the **anode**. Electrons are produced at the cathode in the **filament**.

Most radiographic tubes have two filaments, a large and small one; such tubes are known as double focus tubes. The filaments are tungsten wire coils, which are set into **focusing cups**, Figure 6-2. The focusing cup (see Figures 6-1 and 6-2) is used to direct the flow of electrons. The electrons flow from negative (cathode) to positive (anode) across the tube. The focusing cup surrounds the filament and

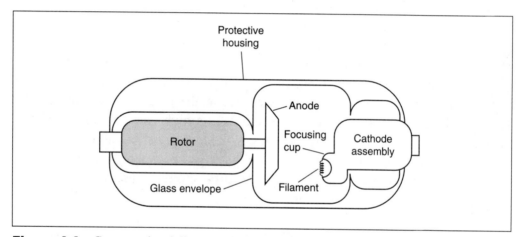

Figure 6-1   Cross-sectional diagram of a typical diagnostic X-ray tube

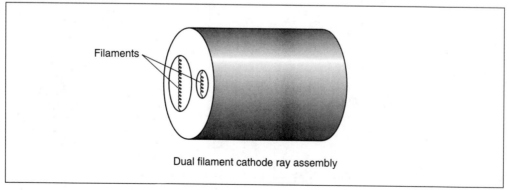

Figure 6-2   Dual filament focusing cup

also has a negative potential, as does the filament (cathode). This combination of negatively charged cathode and negatively charged focusing cup allows the electrons to bombard the positively charged anode (target) in a specific focus area (focus spot size) based on the line focus principle. Otherwise, when the electrons impact the target, they would spread damaging heat over the whole target surface. The filament is heated by a high electrical **filament current**, which is measured in amperes. The current heats the tungsten (wire) and electrons are emitted from the filament in a process called **thermionic emission**. As the current is increased to the filament, the number of emitted electrons is increased. The amount of electrons generated in the tube determines the amount of milliamperes (mA) (or quantity of radiation), which results in the overall blackening on the recorded image. Overall blackening is the density as seen in the recorded image (See Density in Chapter 8). When the electrons are released, they collect in the space around the filament and remain there until electrical force is applied to move them. The force applied to move the electrons is measured in thousands of volts and is called kilovoltage (kV). The kilovoltage is applied through the potential difference across the tube, creating a net negative charge at the filament on the cathode side and a net positive charge at the target on the anode side. The kilovoltage force accelerates the electrons at a high velocity across the gap from the cathode to the anode, where they strike the part of the anode known as the **target**, Figure 6-3. The electron stream that flows between the cathode (negative) and anode (positive) makes up the **tube current**, measured in milliamperes (mA), and is called milliamperage.

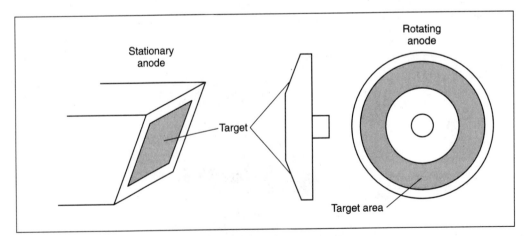

Figure 6-3   Stationary anode *(left)* and rotating anode *(right)*

The electron stream is focused on one part of the anode, called the target. The anode is made of tungsten and may be either a stationary wedge or a rotating disk. Tungsten is used because it has a very high melting point—3370°C and an atomic number (z) of 74 (z = 74). It can therefore withstand much more heat than other metal materials. There is an enormous amount of heat created by the inter-action of electrons in the anode, and tungsten is an excellent material for absorb-ing high degrees of heat. It should be pointed out that the target material's ability to withstand heat affects both the quantity (mAs) of X-rays and the quality (kVp) of the X-ray energy. Increased mAs results in increased quantity, which results in increased blackness on the recorded image. Increased kVp results in increased penetration, with greater efficiency of the radiation penetration. Additionally, as kVp increases, scatter radiation increases. To help dissipate the large volume of heat, however, the anode may be made to rotate so that the heat is spread over the entire surface of the anode during exposure. Some tubes may be constructed with a rhenium-tungsten alloy anode. The combination of rhenium (z = 75) and tung-sten (z = 74) further reduces the heat load and subsequent thermal stress and may reduce the potential for surface roughening, cracking, or pitting. Additionally, the combination increases the efficiency of X-ray projection as well as resistance to the heat-related problems previously mentioned.

When the electrons are flowing at a high rate of speed and are stopped suddenly at the anode and interact with the anode, the production of radiant energy (X rays) occurs. Unfortunately, the kinetic energy is transformed mostly to heat (99 percent) and very little to useful X rays (1 percent), which is what is needed to produce the radiographic image. The cited percentage of heat and X ray produced from the energized tube varies. Most textbooks state that the percent-age of useful X rays produced is between 1 and 2 percent. It is, however, the vast amount of heat production that may result in excessive tube heating.

As the electron stream strikes the anode surface, most of the X rays are pro-jected perpendicular to the electron beam through the window opening (portal exit plane) in the tube housing (Figure 6-1). Tubes that are constructed with anodes that do not rotate have limited exposure capacity (i.e., dental units).

The radiographic tube has essentially been described, but further discussion of certain parts and their principal function is necessary. The tube components are enclosed in a glass envelope from which air has been removed. The tube must have as much gas or air removed as possible. Otherwise, the electrons would collide with gas molecules, thus reducing tube current. Also an evacuated tube has a longer life span and will not burn out as quickly.

A radiographic tube, like an electric light bulb, has a wire filament. A light bulb or an X-ray tube will burn out when the filament evaporates or becomes thinner. This occurs with age or usage when the tube is operated at maximum capacity. The radiographic machine itself is equipped with a double switch on the console (control panel). One switch, called the rotor, is used to heat the filament and to start the anode rotating to bring it up to the proper RPM (e.g., 3,000 or 10,000). The other switch actually makes the exposure. This also maintains control over the exposure. To reduce the amount of filament evaporation and extend the tube life, the rotor switch should only be used when the exposure is ready to be made. The radiographer should not hold the rotor switch on while instructing the patient. The small filament (corresponding to the small focal spot) may burn out faster than the larger one (corresponding to the large focal spot) depending on usage.

THE LINE FOCUS PRINCIPLE

The cathode (negative) side of the tube has been referred to several times. Electrons flow from negative (cathode) toward the positive (anode) side of the tube. The tungsten wire filament is mounted on the cathode in a cup-shaped depression, called the focusing cup, that serves to focus the electron beam on the anode target, Figure 6-4. The **line focus principle** is a result of the electron

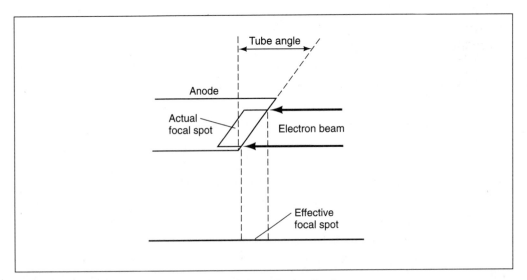

Figure 6-4   The line focus principle and the effective focal spot

stream striking an angled target (i.e., ten degrees, twenty degrees). The part of the anode on which the electron beam impacts is called the **focal spot**. The effect is that of making the resulting X-ray beam smaller than the electron beam. Consequently, when an anode disk with less angle is used along with a small focal spot, the recorded image will have greater detail.

The electrons from the filament actually strike the anode in a rectangular shape, such as 1.0 mm × 3.0 mm, but effectively create an image on a film more square—1.0 mm × 1.0 mm. Thus, the radiographer must understand the difference between the **actual focal spot** and the **effective focal spot**. The size of the effective focal spot is based on 1) the angle of the tube and 2) the size of the filament.

TUBE RATING CHARTS

The purpose of a tube rating chart, Figure 6-5, is to extend the life of a tube and to assure that the tube can withstand the heat created by the workload. There are certain instantaneous ratings that are excessive and can seriously damage or cause a melting point on the tube anode surface. Such considerations include:

1. Never use high kVp on a cold target. The target must be warmed with several low exposures (low kVp, low mAs; i.e., 50kVp 10mA) before making a single high exposure. A tube target will become cold after about an hour of nonuse. Always warm the target when beginning the day's work or when the tube has cooled for a long period.
2. Never use an *excessive* single exposure, even on a warm anode.
3. The number of multiple exposures (e.g., twenty) that may be made at any given time must not exceed the tube's total heat capacity.
4. A radiographic tube that uses a fixed anode—one that does not rotate—is limited in its heat capacity and thus uses lower kVp and mA levels (i.e., dental unit).

Radiographers generally need only be concerned with warming a cold anode and not exceeding a single exposure rate on the anode. Remember, the rules for protecting and properly using a radiographic tube are easily followed through the manufacturer's recommendations included on rating charts that come with the tube purchase.

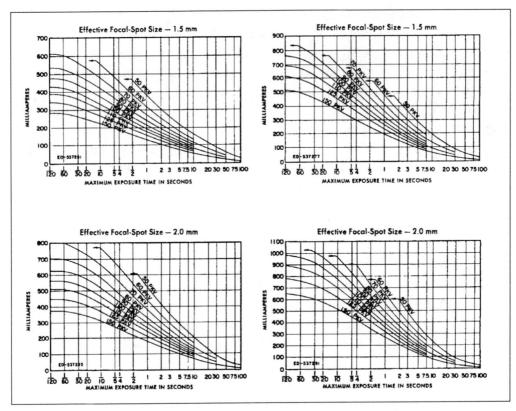

Figure 6-5   Representative tube rating charts for a diagnostic X-ray tube

TUBE HEAT CAPACITY

Tube heat capacity has been referred to several times because the tube's problems are directly related to heat. Tube heat capacity is measured in heat units (HU). Heat units are simply a mathematical combination of exposure factors, kilovoltage (kVp), seconds (s), and milliamperage (mA) written in formula as kVp × s × mA. For detailed discussion about these exposure factors, refer to chapters 5 and 8. For now, let's say that the exposure factors 70 kVp × 1.0 seconds × 100 mA equal 7000 HU. The preceding formula may be used to calculate HU for single phase current. To calculate for 3 phase current, the same formula may be used by factoring in 1.35 for 3 phase, 6 pulse and 1.41 for 3 phase, 12 pulse. Examples follow:

$$1.35 \times 70 \text{ kVp} \times 1.0 \text{ sec.} \times 100 \text{ mA} = 9450 \text{ HU}$$
$$1.41 \times 70 \text{ kVp} \times 1.0 \text{ sec.} \times 100 \text{ mA} = 9870 \text{ HU}$$

Whether or not that number of HU would be more than the heat capacity of a given tube would depend on its total capacity and how much heat in HU had already been applied. Depending on the tube's intended workload, heat units vary from as little as 100,000HU to 400,000HU. It is prudent for the radiographer to know and respect the manufacturer's recommended tube capacity.

REVIEW QUESTIONS

1. The cathode beam of an X-ray tube is the
   a) primary X-ray beam
   b) focused electron beam within the tube
   c) current heating the filament
   d) secondary radiation

2. The target metal used in X-ray tubes should have the following two properties
   a) high atomic number, high melting point
   b) low atomic number, low melting point
   c) low atomic number, high melting point
   d) high atomic number, low melting point

3. The process of boiling off of electrons from a hot, metallic filament is called
   a) Compton scatter
   b) pair production
   c) photoelectric effect
   d) thermionic emission

4. The positive terminal of an X-ray tube is the
   a) cathode
   b) anode
   c) focusing cup
   d) filament

5. The cloud of liberated electrons that remains in the vicinity of the hot filament is called
   a) tube current
   b) filament current
   c) positrons
   d) space charge

6. The negative terminal of an X-ray tube is the
    a) cathode
    b) anode
    c) target
    d) rotor

7. X rays are produced in the
    1) focal spot
    2) anode
    3) target
        a) 1 and 2
        b) 1 and 3
        c) 2 and 3
        d) 1, 2, and 3

8. The effective focal spot
    1. is smaller than the actual focal spot
    2. is on the anode
    3. determines the resolution
        a) 1 and 2
        b) 1 and 3
        c) 2 and 3
        d) 1, 2, and 3

9. A rotating anode
    1. dissipates heat
    2. has a larger target than a fixed anode
    3. is driven by a motor
        a) 1 and 2
        b) 1 and 3
        c) 2 and 3
        d) 1, 2, and 3

10. The tube housing
    1. helps contain scattered X rays
    2. is designed to aid in heat dissipation
    3. contains the glass envelope
        a) 1 and 2
        b) 1 and 3
        c) 2 and 3
        d) 1, 2, and 3

11. The most important component of a radiographic unit with regard to image production is the X-ray tube
    a) true
    b) false
12. The X-ray tube focusing cup has a _____ charge.
    a) positive
    b) negative
13. Heat units may be determined with the following formula:
    a) kVp × S × mA
    b) kVp × mA
    c) kVp × S × 1.41
    d) kVp × mA × 1.35
    e) none of the above
14. The rotating anode is generally made of an alloy material with a high melting point. The following element(s) represent the most efficient material(s) for X-ray production.
    a) gold
    b) tungsten
    c) rhenium-tungsten
    d) a and b
    e) b and c
15. The amount of electrons generated in the X-ray tube determines the _____.
    a) quality
    b) quantity
    c) mA
    d) a and c
    e) b and c

Chapter 7

Imaging Equipment

Chapter Outline

Introduction
Radiographic Equipment
Primary and Secondary Circuits
  Primary Circuit
  Secondary Circuit
Types of Equipment
Accessory Items
  Calipers
  Cassettes

Objectives

Upon completion of the chapter, the student will meet the following objectives by verifying knowledge, facts, and principles presented through oral and written communication at a level deemed competent and will meet the task objectives by demonstrating the specific behavior as identified in the terminal performance objectives of the procedures.

1. Explain permanently installed radiographic equipment and its maintenance.
2. Identify and discuss the various types and purposes of basic radiographic equipment.
3. Discuss the purposes, advantages, and disadvantages of routine and specific radiographic equipment.
4. Describe the purpose and disadvantages of mobile equipment and relate complexity of procedures.
5. Describe accessory equipment and the usage of different types.
6. Demonstrate competence in each task listed below. Refer to the appendix for the individual procedure/performance guides.

   TASKS (See Appendix):
   7-1 Cleaning Radiographic Facilities and Equipment.
   7-2 Operating Radiographic Tables and Consoles.

INTRODUCTION

This chapter deals with the electrical equipment needed to produce the radiographic image. It is important that prospective radiographers possess functional knowledge about the equipment they will use to practice their profession. Knowledge of the basis of the operation of radiographic units provides the radiographer with the background to use the imaging equipment most efficiently.

RADIOGRAPHIC EQUIPMENT

Radiographic equipment is the instrumentation needed for the performance of the tasks associated with radiographic procedures. Generally, we think of the permanently installed equipment—that which is used for either fluoroscopy or radiography, Figure 7-1. However, many items used as accessories in the production of radiographic images (e.g., grid cassettes, compression bands, etc.) are also considered radiographic equipment.

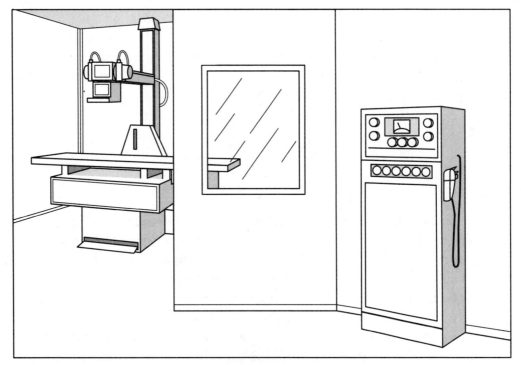

Figure 7-1 Permanently installed radiographic equipment (*Courtesy of GE Medical Systems*)

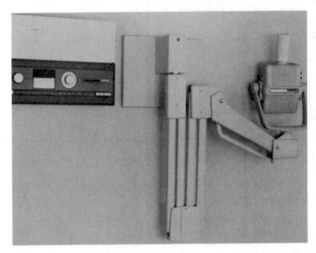

Figure 7-2   Dental x-ray machine used for intraoral radiographs. GX-1000 with Panelipse II Master Control (GENDEX Corporation, Milwaukee, WI). This control panel permits a choice of milliampere rate and kilovoltage in addition to exposure time and can be used for two different tubeheads. *(Courtesy of GENDEX Corporation.)*

The most important component of any radiographic unit is the tube. (The tube was discussed in detail in Chapter 6.) The tube is a rotational or fixed part of a unit that also includes an electrical system and controls for circuits, generators, fuses, and switches. According to its purpose, a piece of equipment may be large, with many different components, or small, like a dental unit that hangs on the wall, Figure 7-2. All equipment must be handled with care and have regular maintenance, quality assurance, and testing to provide reliability.

Radiographic units may be divided into two basic parts: the primary circuit (also called the low-voltage circuit), and the secondary or high-voltage circuit.

PRIMARY AND SECONDARY CIRCUITS

When a radiographic unit is installed, there must be a current source that comes from an outside source. The local utility company is responsible for the main supply of the incoming 110 or 220 volts of alternating current that will be used for any facility. Lines are brought in from outside and connected to a junction box inside, where the radiographic unit control console is connected.

To produce X rays, the line voltage must be controlled and changed to a direct current of many thousands of volts. This is done by the high-voltage transformer. A transformer is an electromagnetic device that will increase or decrease the voltage of alternating current. In an X-ray machine, the high-voltage transformer increases the low voltage of the primary circuit to the high voltage needed by the secondary circuit.

Primary Circuit

The primary circuit begins at the main power switch on the control console of the radiographic unit and leads to the primary coil of the high-tension transformer, Figure 7-3. Major components included in the primary section of the circuit are the autotransformer, kilovolt peak meter, voltage compensator, filament circuit, circuit breaker, and timers.

Autotransformer. This special type of transformer is used with the major and minor kVp selectors to provide a means to vary the voltage magnitude, through a step-up transformer and a step-down transformer. A step-up transformer increases voltage and decreases current. A step-down transformer decreases voltage and increases current.

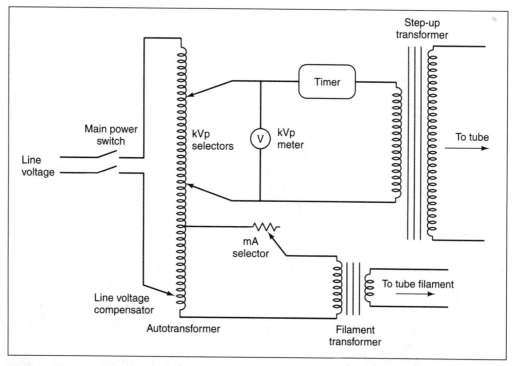

Figure 7-3 Schematic diagram of the primary side of an X-ray machine circuit

Kilovolt Peak Meter. This meter is connected to the autotransformer. Its function is to display the potential difference in kilovolts going to the high-voltage transformer.

Line Voltage Compensator. This component is connected across or in parallel with the primary circuit to the autotransformer. Its function is to increase or decrease the line voltage if there is a drop or surge in the line voltage. Any change in input voltage will cause a change in output of radiation. Automatic line-voltage compensators are included in modern radiographic units.

Filament Circuit. The filament circuit is connected to the autotransformer. Its function is to supply current to the filament of the radiographic tube. The circuit supplies lower voltage and higher current by means of a step-down transformer, which is controlled by a rheostat or variable resistor.

Circuit Breaker. This is a protective device used to automatically terminate the current in the event that predetermined values are exceeded, i.e., excessive exposure or too much current from the line source. The breaker may be reset mechanically with a switch. If exposure factors cut off the breaker, then lower settings must be selected.

Timers. Duration of exposure time is controlled by a switch in the timing circuit. The switch, which is built into the electrical circuit, will remain closed for the length of time selected by the radiographer at the control console or panel. Several types of exposure-timing devices are commonly used.

1. *Synchronous timers*: A synchronous timer is controlled and driven by an electrical synchronous motor. It is not generally used because it is not reliable and has limited exposure-time range. Exposure times are not usually accurate for shorter than 1/60 of a second.
2. *Electronic timers*:
   Impulse—A precise timing circuit that operates with an alternating current. The circuit is energized to variable time intervals, from milliseconds to seconds. It is accurate and may be used for rapid film production.
   mAs—A more specific electronic timer is used to control and terminate the time when the correct mAs is reached. This type of mAs timer is protection for tube current.
3. *Automatic timers*: A timing device that automatically terminates the exposure when the correct amount of radiation (density) has reached the film. The accu-

racy of this device depends on carefully positioning the anatomical part being radiographed correctly to the sensing element of the timing device.

Automatic exposure-control devices are categorized as phototimer and ionization chamber.

Phototimer utilizes a light-sensitive photomultiplier tube placed behind a fluorescent screen. The fluorescent screen, placed in front of or behind the film, produces light from radiation transmitted through the film. The light is picked up by the photomultiplier tube which terminates the exposure, after a predetermined charge that corresponds to the density of the film is reached. The amount of screen fluorescence (intensity) is directly proportional to the amount of radiation (intensity) that reaches the film.

Ionization chamber utilizes a chamber located between the patient and the film. This chamber measures the amount of radiation reaching the film and shuts off the exposure at a predetermined setting.

Timer Tests. Two types of devices are used for testing the accuracy of timers. One is a simple manual spinning top designed to test single phase current (see Figure 7-4). Single phase units are less common today because most radiology departments or offices have advanced, full-wave rectification radiographic units that utilize 3-phase current. This type of current should be tested with an electric meter. The device used for single phase units is placed on top of a film cassette

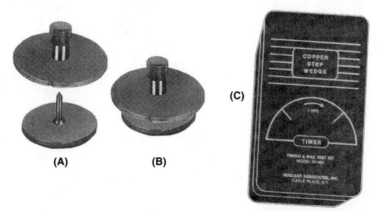

Figure 7-4 (A) A spin top is used to measure timer accuracy of single-phase equipment. A brass disc base with a spindle at its center, and the top with a small hole near its edge is exhibited. The spin top, which is easily rotated, is shown in (B). (C) A timer and mAs tester. This device may be used for single-phase, as well as three-phase radiographic equipment. It is a synchronous rotator-slit timer tester, and is used for checking timer accuracy and mAs uniformity. The manufacturer provides directions for appropriate use of the timing and mAs device.

and manually rotated (like a spinning top) not too fast or too slow. The single opening on the disk will show up on the film as dots that represent electrical current flow for 60-cycle current at 120 impulses per second. In order to determine the number of dots to be seen on the film, the exposure timer should be set for a given time and the time divided into 120; e.g., 0.1/120 = 12 dots.

Electric mAs meters used for testing 3-phase current are a little more involved because the dots overlap as a result of multiple electrical impulses (see Figure 7-4). This type of device records an arc on the film. The meter is placed on the film cassette and exposed at a given time. The resulting exposure will show an arc of overlapped dots. The degree of the arc must be measured with a protractor provided with the meter. The degree of the arc is divided into the number of impulses; e.g., 90°/360 = 0.4. Instructions for using the mAs meters generally come with the individual device.

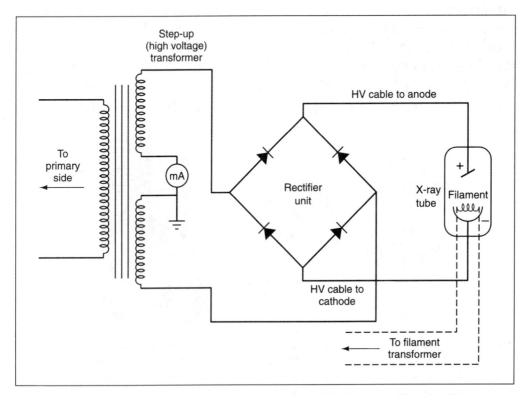

Figure 7-5   Schematic diagram of the secondary side of an X-ray machine circuit

Secondary Circuit

The high-voltage, secondary circuit begins with the secondary coil of the step-up transformer (see Figure 7-5). It also includes the milliameter (mA), milliampere second meter (mAs), rectifiers, high-voltage cables and radiographic tube. All components of the secondary circuit are immersed in oil for purposes of electrical insulation and cooling in a separate section away from the radiographic unit console.

High-Voltage Transformer. The step-up, or high-voltage transformer consists of two iron coils wrapped with windings of electrical wire. The coil on the low-voltage side, carrying the current from the primary circuit, is called the primary coil. The coil on the high-voltage side carries the stepped-up, or increased voltage to the secondary circuit and is called the secondary coil.

Milliameter (mA). The mA meter is used to measure the current in milliamperes flowing through the radiographic tube. It is connected in series with the high-voltage circuit.

Rectifiers. Rectifiers are used to change alternating current to direct current, or current flowing in one direction, Figure 7-6A and B. Alternating current is used in the primary circuit for two reasons: 1) it is the type of electricity supplied by the electrical utility, and 2) transformers will only work on alternating current. However, direct current is necessary to operate the radiographic tube so that electrons can be produced and kept flowing in one direction. Any reverse or change in current flow would cease electron production and could damage the tube. Rectification is controlled in modern equipment by devices called *diodes*. Modern radiographic equipment uses solid-state, silicone diode rectifiers to convert alternating current to direct current.

Two types of rectification are used in diagnostic radiology X-ray machines:

1. *Half-wave rectification*, Figure 7-6A. This type of rectification is used where current is directed by one or two diodes. Negative voltage is suppressed so that the flow of current is only utilized during the positive flow of alternating current. It is also called impulse current because one cycle of alternating current is applied.
2. *Full-wave rectification*, Figure 7-6B. This type of rectification is used in most radiographic units because it is the most efficient. It uses four diodes so that both the positive and negative impulses are used. There is a constant flow of positive current in one direction.

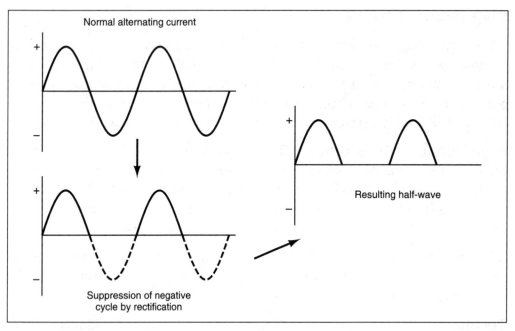

Figure 7-6A   Half-wave rectification of normal alternating current and the resulting waveform

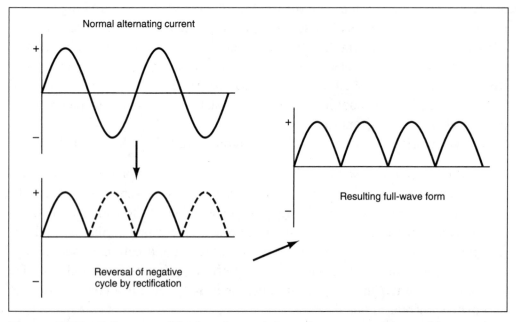

Figure 7-6B   Full-wave rectification of normal alternating current and the resulting waveform

High-Voltage Cables. Two large cables are used to connect the radiographic tube to the high-voltage generator. One cable is attached to the cathode side of the tube; the other is connected to the anode side of the tube. The cables are designed to prevent any electrical hazard, such as arcing over of current flow from one terminal to the other.

Radiographic Tube. This component is the most important part of the radiographic unit. It is the component that creates the electrons that are used to produce the X rays that are the basis for radiographic images. Again, the tube is described in detail in Chapter 6.

TYPES OF EQUIPMENT

Various types of units, either combined radiographic and fluoroscopic units (RF) or radiographic units only, may be found where radiographic images are produced. They may be installed for general or specific examination purposes, e.g., chest unit or head unit. In addition to installed units, there are portable units, used principally at the bedside. Important items of information to learn and remember about all radiographic units are:

1. *The electrical capacity of the unit in terms of milliamperage and kilovoltage.* Unless a radiographer is working with outdated equipment, a standard unit may have exposure ratings of from 100 to 1200 mA, kVp settings up to 150, and a dual focus tube (large and small focal spots). Other exposure factors include various time settings ranging from milliseconds to several whole seconds, i.e., $1/360$–10 seconds, although radiographs are generally made at fractions of seconds.

2. *The limitation of any unit, especially portables.* In regard to portables, although the radiographer today is so concerned with limitation of exposure, the degree of equipment maneuverability is very important. That is, portable radiography may be complex when the patient's condition is unstable or body position must be maintained, as in orthopedic traction. Extensive orthopedic traction for trauma patients usually requires an experienced radiographer's judgment for making films. Some specific units, such as head units, have limitations that restrict examining the patient who is either sitting or lying on a stretcher and cannot be moved. If the head unit is placed in a tight area or the radiographer does not understand its maneuverability, a head unit may become limited to use with the sitting position only.

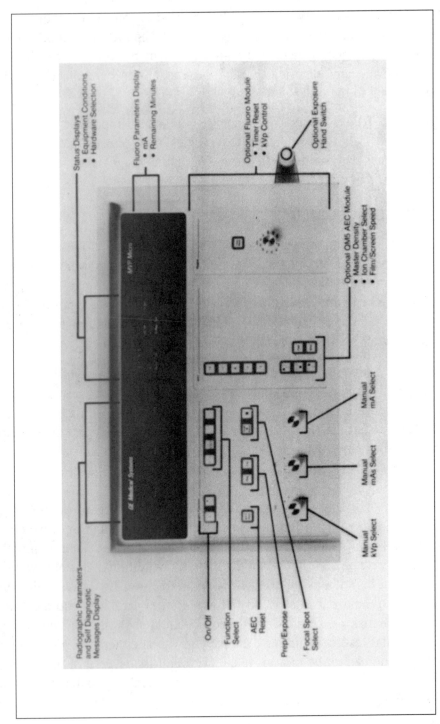

Figure 7-7 The control console of a diagnostic X-ray machine *(Courtesy of GE Medical Systems)*

3. *The purpose and combinations of exposure factors—the mA, time(s), and kVp selections.* The way in which all exposure factors affect the visible image must be clear to the radiographer. The function of all switches and meters on the control panel must be understood, Figure 7-7.
4. *The purpose and effectiveness of radiographic accessory items.* The way in which accessory items aid in the production or enhancement of the radiographic image is essential knowledge for the radiographer.

ACCESSORY ITEMS

Radiography uses numerous accessory items. Some may be unique to a particular radiographic procedure, such as those used in CT, MRI, or ultrasound. The most common items are cassettes, grid cassettes, calipers, film holders, film markers, film printers, compression bands, tape, and sponges. These items are generally found in any radiographic room. Although most are described and their uses explained in Chapters 8 and 9, calipers and cassettes are discussed in this chapter.

Calipers

A caliper is a measuring device, used in radiography to measure the volume of tissue thickness of a body part. Tissue volume is a variable in exposure technique that must be accounted for in image production. It is a mistake to believe that one can simply and accurately visually judge tissue volume. Beyond a certain point, quality begins to suffer when one attempts to "guess" what every set of technical factors will be through visual estimation only. Moreover, it may often be useful for the radiographer measuring tissue volume with the caliper to be aware that tone and texture of tissues may be determined through touch. These discoveries, of course, cannot be made if one never measures tissue. Thus, we can see the deception of assuming exposure latitude. Exposure latitude allows for gradual margin of error in radiographic quality within certain kVp measurement ranges. An important advantage of measuring tissue volume is consistency of exposure techniques. The same patient may be measured at different times by different people, but the result should be the same, thus reflecting equal exposure factors. It does not take into account conditions, such as ascites (abdominal fluid), where exposure must be manipulated to maintain equal radiographic quality in density and contrast. The effect of tissue measurement may become less critical when some exposure factors are standardized and technique charts are developed on the basis of one-centimeter variations of tissue thickness. The radiographer may be able to visually evaluate tissue thickness by judging the distance between two lines that measure one centimeter.

To place the caliper properly, the (horizontal) sliding part of the device must be parallel to the base of the device and the vertical part must remain perpendicular to the base. The sliding part must not be pushed tightly against the tissue; it should be allowed to rest evenly along the part being measured. Measurement is always taken along the imaginary line where the central ray traverses the body part and at the same angle as the central ray. Extreme differences or variations in the part to be radiographed should be compensated by determining an average thickness within the total area of the part.

Automation of film processing and the use of faster imaging materials and exposure times only increase the essential need for the radiographer to determine exposure variables accurately. Tissue thickness and volume therefore must be taken into account no matter how exposure factors are determined.

Cassettes

A cassette is used to provide mechanical support and protection for the film and contains intensifying screens. Cassettes must be lightweight as well as light-proof, Figure 7-8.

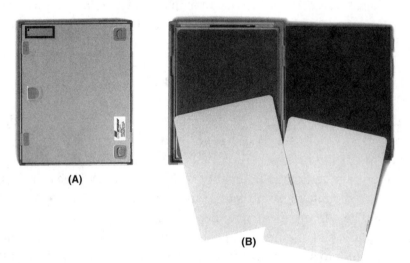

(A)

(B)

Figure 7-8   (A) A closed image receptor (X-ray cassette) used to hold the film. (B) The receptor is opened and shows the screens for the receptor. The front and back screens would be mounted inside the receptor where the film would be placed between them when used to record the image. The purpose of screens is to intensify the action of radiation. *(Courtesy of GE Medical Systems)*

Cassette fronts are made of material that offers almost no filtration to the passage of radiation. Because absorption of moisture may occur and cause expansion and contraction with temperature extremes, warping can result. Materials generally used in construction are: 1) a plastic that will absorb moisture but is radiolucent and 2) a metal alloy such as aluminum or magnesium.

Cassette backs are made of metal, aluminum, or steel. A thin sheet of foil may be attached to the inner side of the back of the cassette to prevent radiation from being scattered back through the cassette to fog film. In the case of photo-timed exposures, unnecessarily long exposures may result unless the photo-tube sensitivity is increased to sufficiently compensate for lead backing in the cassette.

REVIEW QUESTIONS

1. Rectification is a process that changes
   a) direct current to alternating current
   b) alternating current to direct current
   c) high-voltage direct current to low-voltage direct current
   d) high-voltage alternating current to low-voltage alternating current

2. Self-rectification in an X-ray circuit leads to a voltage wave that is the same as
   a) full-wave
   b) half-wave
   c) direct current
   d) two of the above

3. Which of the following is found in the filament circuit?
   a) step-up transformer
   b) step-down transformer
   c) target
   d) exposure timer

4. Which of the following devices would be located between the secondary coil of the high-voltage transformer and the X-ray tube?
   a) rheostat (milliampere selector)
   b) rectifier
   c) autotransformer
   d) filament transformer

5. The function of the filament circuit is to
   a) supply low-voltage current to the anode
   b) supply high-voltage current to the filament
   c) supply low-voltage current to the filament
   d) supply high-voltage current to the autotransformer

6. Which of the following devices is found in the primary circuit?
   a) rectifier circuit
   b) X-ray tube
   c) autotransformer
   d) filament

7. Which type of X-ray timer terminates the exposure when a fluorescent screen produces light from the X rays?
   a) synchronous
   b) impulse
   c) mAs
   d) phototimer

8. Another name for a rectifier is
   a) autotransformer
   b) diode
   c) filament
   d) voltmeter

9. A device used to measure thickness of a body part is a
   a) caliper
   b) meter stick
   c) yard stick
   d) tape measure

10. Cassettes
    1. provide mechanical support for the film
    2. contain intensifying screens
    3. must be light proof
       a) 1 and 2
       b) 1 and 3
       c) 2 and 3
       d) 1, 2, and 3

11. The single most significant component of the radiographic unit is
    a) step-up transformer
    b) half-wave rectifier
    c) tube
    d) none of the above
12. Devices used for testing the accuracy of electrical timers are called
    a) stop watches
    b) manual spinning tops
    c) electric mAs meters
    d) c and d

Chapter **8**

Fundamentals of Radiographic Exposure

Chapter Outline

Objectives

Upon completion of the chapter, the student will meet the following objectives by verifying knowledge of the facts and principles presented through oral and written communication at a level deemed competent.

1. Differentiate between the photographic and geometric properties related to the radiographic image.
2. Define and explain radiographic density as it relates to photographic properties of the radiographic image.

3. Define and explain radiographic contrast as it relates to photographic properties of the radiographic image.
4. Define other types of contrast: subject contrast, film contrast.
5. Define exposure latitude and kilovoltage ranges.
6. Explain what recorded detail means in the visible image.
7. Describe how mA, kVp, time, SID, and heel effect control and affect density and contrast in the radiographic image.
8. Explain the effect of motion on the formation of the radiographic image.
9. Explain the effect of magnification on the formation of the radiographic image.
10. Explain the effect of distortion on the formation of the radiographic image.
11. Given appropriate information, explain how to calculate exposure factors mA, time, kVp, and SID and their collective photographic effect.

INTRODUCTION

In this chapter the student will learn how to manipulate exposure factors according to their interactive effect on the radiographic image. Standardization of radiographic exposure factors, although theoretically based, must be understood in the application of day-to-day radiography. More importantly, the student must understand exposure latitude and how it provides a margin of error which varies depending on mathematical ranges of exposure factors (mA, time, kVp, SID). The quality of the visible radiographic image depends largely on the perception of the viewer. However, with a solid background in the knowledge of human anatomy and an understanding of the technical factors that create a radiographic image, the health professional is able to evaluate the image in discipline-specific terms.

IMAGE PRODUCTION

A radiograph is produced from X rays passing through a patient's body and interacting with the emulsion (surface) of a radiographic film. The finished radiograph is expected to provide a quality diagnostic image of the body part adjacent to the film. The image comprises the outlines and densities of the body part it represents (e.g., stomach, lungs). When processed with appropriate chemicals, the film emulsion yields a radiograph that, when placed on an illuminated light source (viewbox), provides visual information from which the physician can make a radiographic diagnosis.

TABLE 8-1 ▪ Image Interpretation Areas

PHOTOGRAPHIC PROPERTIES	GEOMETRIC PROPERTIES
Density	Recorded Detail
Contrast	Distortion
	Magnification

A diagnostic quality radiograph should have adequate density (blackness), good contrast (range of gray shades), clear recorded detail (definition and resolution), and no visual distortion or magnification (size and shape) of the anatomy being examined. A physician interprets the anatomy in a radiograph based on visual properties. These properties can be categorized into two areas: density and contrast (categorized as photographic properties) and the recorded detail and absence of distortion and magnification (categorized as geometric properties). Table 8-1 summarizes the general parameters for interpreting radiographs. Each of the properties will be discussed further in the chapter.

EXPOSURE FACTORS

Production of the visible radiographic image is controlled by the following exposure factors: milliamperage (mA), time, kilovoltage peak (kVp), and source-to-image distance (SID). However, other factors—heel effect, tube alignment to the film and body part, object-film distance, tissue thickness/pathology, screen selection, collimation and beam filters, fog, and film processing—also influence image production.

Exposure factors and other technical considerations will be discussed in relation to their effect on the image by photographic or geometric consequence. For the sake of simplicity, henceforth mA, time, kVp, and SID will be referred to as factors.

PHOTOGRAPHIC FACTORS

The two major photographic factors of the image are 1) *density* and 2) *contrast*.

Density

Density is seen as the overall blackness of the total image. Density is controlled by *milliamperage-seconds* (mAs)—it represents the quantity of radiation being produced for a certain length of time in an energized radiographic tube (as described in Chapter 6). The mAs to be used during any given radiographic exposure, i.e., 100 mA, 200 mA, 300 mA, is set by the radiographer at the control console of the radiographic unit, Figure 8-1A and B. The density of the radiograph is directly proportional to the amount of mA used for exposure and length of time the exposure is delivered (referred to as mAs setting). A good principle to remember is that, proportionally, 200 mA at 1.0 seconds will produce twice as much density on a film as will 100 mA at 1.0 seconds. Higher mA selections will increase the production of electrons inside the tube (hence, quantity of radiation). Therefore, as more electrons are produced, more radiation reaches the film and more blackness or density will be seen on the film. Density is directly proportional to mA and time. If the mA is doubled, the quantity of radiation will double. If the time is doubled, the quantity of radiation will double. Both mA and time (mAs) have a direct effect on the degree of film darkening (density).

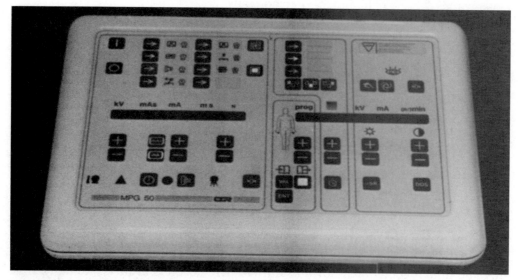

Figure 8-1A The control console is a modern, computerized panel. Only the exposure factors that have been selected are shown on the panel. Older machines may still show individual mA stations and the time (seconds) dial selector. *(Reprinted courtesy of Eastman Kodak Company)*

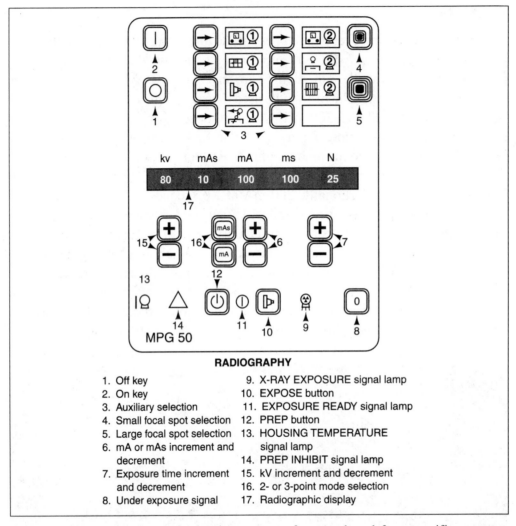

Figure 8-1B Control console showing exposure factors selected for a specific exposure. Controls are defined in the key.

Time and Density. Time is a factor of duration. It expresses the length of time that electrons (mA) are produced in the tube. As previously indicated, mA and time together are known as milliampere-seconds or mAs. Actually, time indicates how long a given amount of mA will last. In other words, milliamperes x time (seconds) = milliampere second (mAs). For example:

$$300 \text{ mA} \times 0.1 \text{ sec} = 30 \text{ mAs}.$$

The quantity of radiation, therefore, must be stated as mAs for four reasons: 1) mAs indicates quantity of radiation and how long the exposure lasted; 2) dosage is a product of mAs (e.g., a 300 mA selection and a time of one second would produce 300 mAs); 3) doubling the time has the same effect as doubling the mA (300 mA × 2 sec = 600 mAs; the quantity of radiation doubles and density or visible blackness in the recorded image doubles); 4) the relationship between mA x T should remain constant during repeated exposures as long as the radiation output is consistent and the generating equipment has been properly calibrated by a company service representative.

The fourth factor above is related to the *Reciprocity Law*. This law means that any combination of mA x T factors that are equivalent mAs should produce the same amount of density. See the following example for further elaboration.

mA	TIME (s)	CALCULATION	mAs
50	$\frac{1}{5}$ sec.	50 × $\frac{1}{5}$ sec. =	10 mAs
100	$\frac{1}{10}$ sec.	100 × $\frac{1}{10}$ sec. =	10 mAs
200	$\frac{1}{20}$ sec.	200 × $\frac{1}{20}$ sec. =	10 mAs
300	$\frac{1}{30}$ sec.	300 × $\frac{1}{30}$ sec. =	10 mAs

All of the above combinations should produce the same amount of density in the image (overall blackness). Thus, if a faster time is needed to avoid motion, mA and time may be changed according to the equation in the example.

Because time is a factor of duration, it is important to always identify the fastest exposure time compatible with other exposure factors (mA, kVp, SID) to avoid capturing any patient or organ motion in the recorded image.

Factors that control the mAs selection are: 1) the size of the focal spot to be used and 2) the amount of exposure time needed. Focal spots are the primary factor controlling recorded detail (a geometric property). However, their ability to withstand heat units inside the tube is critical to how much mAs may be applied for a given technique. Other factors will be discussed in this chapter in topics related to recorded detail (subtopic of Geometric Factors) and to motion (subtopic of Distortion and Magnification). Smaller focal-spot (filament) size in the tube results in sharper recorded detail of the anatomy seen in a radiographic image. For this reason, whenever practical, a smaller focal-spot size should be used. However, if the anatomy being radiographed is thick (large tissue volume, above 12 cm), a larger focal-spot size must be used due to the increased production of internal tube heat (see Chapter 6). Thus, a disadvantage of the smaller focal-spot size is that it cannot tolerate the heat generated with the long or increased exposure time that may be required for thick body parts. The lower mA stations (i.e., 100 mA, 200 mA, and 300 mA) reflect a smaller focal spot. Larger focal-spot sizes are automatically switched on in the generator circuitry with larger mA selections (400 mA, 500 mA, 800 mA, and higher). Combinations of the formula $mA \times T = mAs$ follow.

SMALL FOCAL SPOT

$300 \text{ mA} \times 0.10 \text{ T} = 30 \text{ mAs}$

$300 \text{ mA} \times 0.5 \text{ T} = 150 \text{ mAs}$

LARGE FOCAL SPOT

$600 \text{ mA} \times 0.05 \text{ T} = 30 \text{ mAs}$

$600 \text{ mA} \times 0.25 \text{ T} = 150 \text{ mAs}$

The examples show that $mA \times T$ may be used to achieve the same density on the recorded image using different focal-spot sizes. This factor is also related to the Reciprocity Law referred to on page 159 (see related examples).

The mA stations and their related focal-spot sizes vary with equipment and the particular heat unit capacity (HU) of the specific manufacturer's radiographic tube, Table 8-2.

Heat unit (HU) capacity has been discussed in Chapter 6; however, subject matter is reiterated here for emphasis. The formula for determining HU capacity is:

$$mA \times T \times kVp$$

For example:

$$300 \text{ mA} \times 1 \text{ sec} \times 80 \text{ kVp} = 2400 \text{ HU}$$

For 3-phase units (6 pulse and 12 pulse), the formulas are:

---

6 pulse: $1.35 \times 300 \text{ mA} \times 1.0 \text{ sec} \times 80 \text{ kVp} = 32,400$

12 pulse: $1.41 \times 300 \text{ mA} \times 1.0 \text{ sec} \times 80 \text{ kVp} = 33,840$

TABLE 8-2 ▪ Advantages/Disadvantages of Small and Large Focal Spots

FOCAL-SPOT SIZE (FSS)	ADVANTAGES	DISADVANTAGES
Smaller Focal Spot (100, 200, 300 mA stations)	Results in greater recorded detail of image.	Longer (slower) exposure time may result in patient motion. Focal spot cannot tolerate heat generated by a long exposure time.
Larger Focal Spot (400, 500, 800 mA stations)	Shorter (faster) exposure time minimizes risk of patient motion. Focal spot can tolerate increased heat generated by longer exposure times.	Results in loss of recorded detail of image.

If the total tube capacity is 300,000 HU, then the exposure cited in the first example would use only a small portion (0.08%) of the total capacity. The tube therefore could still withstand much more heat, which would allow several more exposures within the same range.

Other factors that interact to change the direct effect of density are *kVp*, *SID*, *heel effect*, *film processing*, and *fog*.

Quantity of radiation for technique charts may be determined by trial and error using various combinations of mA × T on a phantom or device that represents the equivalency of human body structure. *Never use real human subjects* to establish technique factors. Once the average adult quantity of radiation has been established for a given part of the body, e.g., head or chest, it is seldom necessary to adjust the mA. Only the time factor and sometimes the kilovoltage will need to be adjusted for various thickness ranges of anatomical structures. Table 8-3 shows examples of time variations.

TABLE 8-3 ▪ Examples of Time Variations for Average Adult Chest

CHEST	mA	cm MEASUREMENT	T	mAs
	300	Small 15–18	$\frac{1}{30}$	10
	300	Medium 19–22	$\frac{1}{15}$	20
	300	Large 25–32	$\frac{1}{10}$	30

Note: The chart shows how the time can be adjusted to accommodate various chest-size ranges without changing the mA. However, these calculations may not be appropriate for a given radiographic unit.

kVp and Density. kVp controls contrast. It does, however, affect density in two ways. As kVp is increased, the stream of electrons in the tube moves more efficiently across the tube and results in increased part penetration (discussed later with kVp). A second effect is that as kVp is increased, more radiation energy is produced, resulting in more scattered radiation, which increases density to the film (recorded image). This can be controlled by use of a grid (discussed under Accessories).

Distance and Density. Distance, or source-to-image distance (SID), has a significant influence on density. The effect of distance on density (SID) obeys the *inverse square law*, Figure 8-2. Understanding the concept of the inverse square law is necessary because it relates to density, radiation intensity, and radiation dosage. The inverse square law states: *The intensity of radiation is inversely proportional to the square of the distance.* That is, if forty inches SID is increased to eighty inches SID, the radiation beam spreads over an area four times greater and its intensity diminishes by a factor of four. A change in distance (SID) requires a new mAs value in order to obtain the same amount of density on the radiograph. If the SID is changed to eighty inches from forty inches, a new mAs value is needed to prevent film density from being very light or underexposed. In order to obtain the same amount of density at eighty inches, more initial radiation exposure is required as based on the inverse square law. The following formula may be applied:

$$\frac{mAs_1}{mAs_2} = \frac{D_2^2}{D_1^2}$$

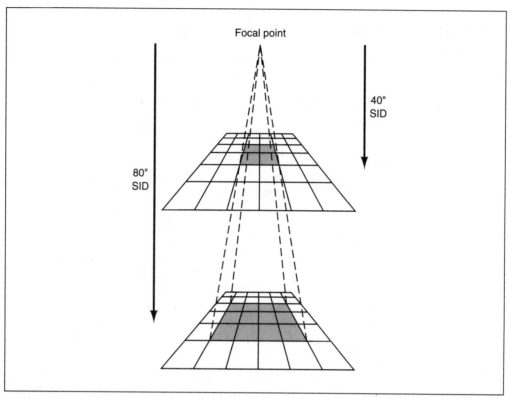

Figure 8-2 At forty inches, a four-square area represents the SID spread. At eighty inches, twice the distance, a sixteen-square area represents the SID and shows increased spread for the same quantity of radiation.

Where: mAs_1 = original mAs

mAs_2 = new mAs

D_2^2 = original distance squared

D_1^2 = new distance squared

The above formula expresses an inverse relationship between SID changes and new mAs. Therefore, making any change in the SID requires a change in milliamperage or time (mAs). A change from forty inches to eighty inches SID is the same as reducing the radiation intensity four times. Thus, the amount of density reduction seen in the image occurs because the intensity of the radiation beam has been attenuated or thinned out over four times more area when twice the distance is used. See Table 8-4 for examples of the effect of the inverse square law.

TABLE 8-4 ▪ Examples Based on Use of the Inverse Square Law

A INCREASE IN SID (Doubled)				B DECREASE IN SID (Halved)			
SID	mAs	SID	mAs	SID	mAs	SID	mAs
40	30	80	120	40	30	20	7.5

$$\frac{30 \text{ mAs}}{x} = \frac{80^2 \text{ SID}}{40^2}$$

$$\frac{30 \text{ mAs}}{x} = \frac{20^2 \text{ SID}}{40^2}$$

$$\frac{30 \text{ mAs}}{x} = \frac{6400 \text{ SID}}{1600}$$

$$\frac{30 \text{ mAs}}{x} = \frac{400 \text{ SID}}{1600}$$

$$6400x = 48000$$

$$400x = 48000$$

$$x = 7.5 \text{ mAs}$$

$$x = 120 \text{ mAs}$$

Note: Using the inverse square law formula. Column A shows the "4 times" decrease in mAs that would result if the SID were doubled from 40 to 80, as seen in Figure 8-2. There would be a corresponding decrease in density in the recorded image, and the image would be underexposed. Column B shows the "4 times" increase in mAs that would result if the SID were halved from 40 to 20. This would result in a corresponding increase in density in the recorded image, and the image would be greatly overexposed.

Simply put, the radiation beam diverges and proceeds in a straight path (lines). The area covered becomes increasingly larger with lessened intensity as the beam of radiation travels a greater distance from the source. To produce a given density at a different distance, it is necessary to vary the exposure inversely with the square of the distance. The exposure area in Figure 8-2 has increased four times from 40 inches to 80 inches.

Heel Effect and Density.   Heel effect is a phenomenon related to the structure of the radiographic tube, i.e., the tube's target (anode) angle. Figure 8-3 shows the long axis of the tube and how the radiation beam is emitted from the focal spot. The radiation intensity diminishes along a line parallel with the long axis of the tube, i.e., the heel effect. As shown in Figure 8-3A, the intensity of the

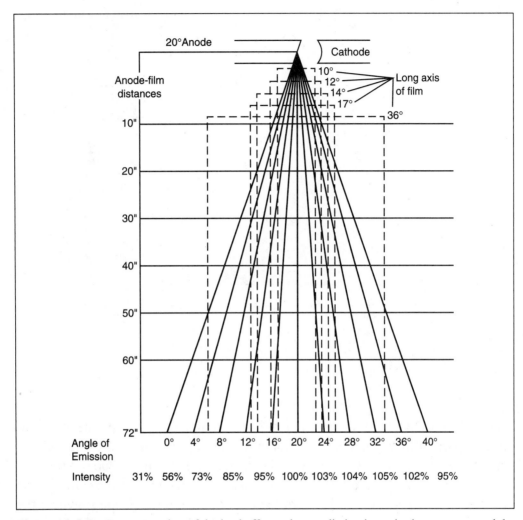

Figure 8-3A Representation of the heel effect, where radiation intensity increases toward the cathode end of the tube

exposure increases toward the cathode (filament) side of the tube while it decreases toward the anode (target) side of the tube as a result of the target angle. This creates more radiation to be emitted at the cathode side of the tube. The effect is more pronounced in tubes with steeper target angles (10 degrees) than in tubes with greater target angles (20 degrees), Figure 8-3B. The heel effect should be utilized to equalize the exposure distribution over various-thickness tissue densities.

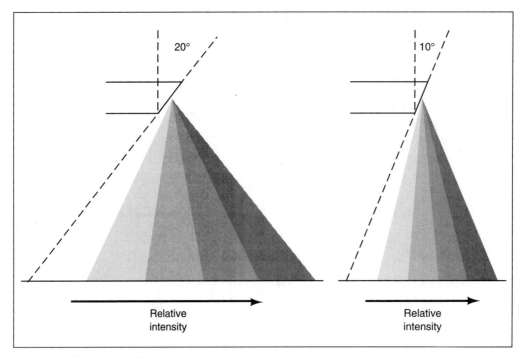

Figure 8-3B   Heel effect

The rule should be to align the long axis of the tube parallel with the longer or broader portion of the anatomical structure being examined so that the cathode side of the tube is directed over the thicker part of the structure. One example for proper tube alignment is radiographic examination of the femur. The cathode side of the tube should be directed toward the hip region and the anode side over the knee region so that the more intense radiation will pass through the adjacent thicker upper femoral area. Another example is the examination of the lower leg. The cathode side should be directed toward the knee thickness or proximal leg to balance radiation distribution. A final example is a lateral lumbar spine. The cathode side of the tube should be directed over the upper pelvic region.

Film Fog and Density.   Density may also be affected by film fog, which is unwanted density that makes it difficult to visualize structures on the radiograph. Film fog may be caused by age (old film), light (result is total blackening of film emulsion), scattered radiation exposure, or improper film development. In order to prevent or reduce film fog, the darkroom must be lightproof. The darkroom safelight should be well-positioned and maintained. Film must be used according to its expiration date. Radiographic film must be processed properly, and unused film should be stored in a lead-lined room or container. Any change in processing time or temperature will quickly affect density in a radiograph. Chapter 9 discusses in more detail why time and temperature must remain constant.

Artifacts are foreign or unwanted marks that show up on a radiograph because of improper film handling, improper processing, or faulty equipment. Artifacts can result in a change (either an increase or a decrease) in film density, usually in a particular area of the image.

Contrast

Contrast is the second major photographic factor. There are three types of contrast: radiographic, subject, and film. Each will be discussed as to its role in a diagnostic quality radiograph.

Radiographic contrast results from the distribution of black metallic silver in the film emulsion and is directly controlled by the penetrating effects of kilovoltage. Radiographic contrast is visualized in the image as gray tones or degrees of gray that reveal the differences between body organs or tissues. Contrast enhances information. If no contrast can be seen between organs, then very little information may be visible in the radiographic image. An excellent example of this phenomena in human anatomy is an obese abdomen where the internal organs appear as equal in tissue thickness and therefore density because of fat content. It is like looking for a white goose in a snow storm. Contrast is controlled by the kilovoltage or, more technically, the quality of energy or wavelength (short or long). You may want to refer to the chapter on physics, Chapter 5.

A variety of long and short wavelengths (low and high energies) will demonstrate a range of shades from black to gray to white (gray tones) and their density differences. The differences are easily seen in the structures visible in the radiographic image. In the blacker portion of a radiograph, the visible structures will have absorbed *less* radiation, and the whiter portion of the visible structures will have absorbed *more* radiation. This means that the whiter structures have greater tissue density.

Radiographic contrast is generally referred to as the overall contrast seen in the image. It includes long-scale (more gray tones) contrast and short-scale (more black and white tones) contrast. Radiation of higher energy (shorter wavelength), 70 kVp or more, will produce long-scale contrast with many gray tones,

Figure 8-4A. Additionally, tissues having little difference in thickness or density will appear as images with flat gray tones. If there are large differences in the thickness of body structures, e.g., bone vs. soft tissue, or if 70 kilovoltage and lower is used, short-scale contrast with more pronounced black and white tones will be produced, Figure 8-4B. Much of the radiographic image contrast is influenced by *subject contrast* and *film contrast*.

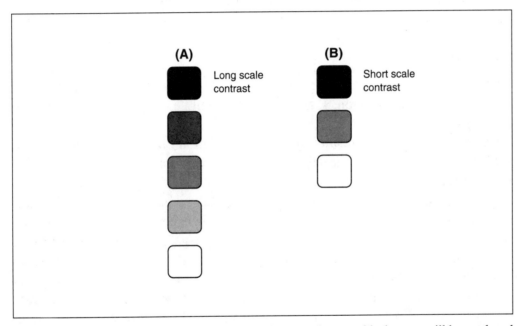

Figure 8-4   A) In long-scale contrast, several degrees of gray to black tones will be produced in the image with higher kVp ranges, i.e., above 70 kVp; B) In short-scale contrast, the range of gray tones is more abrupt from white to black. Fewer gray tones will be seen in the image. Short-scale contrast is produced at lower kVp ranges, i.e., below 70 kVp.

Subject contrast depends on how much the radiation beam is attenuated or spreads out as it enters, passes through, and exits the various structures within the body. This is what is known as an *aerial image*, which is created by the absorption of radiation in various percentages by different tissue thicknesses, Figure 8-5. Bone will absorb more radiation than soft tissue, but this may vary greatly depending on tissue density, age, disease, or other conditions where structure may change or be complex.

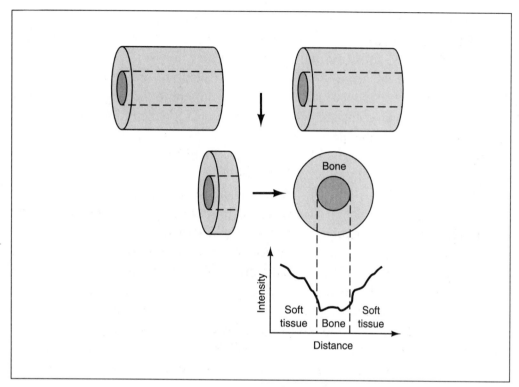

Figure 8-5 Aerial image

Film contrast is inherent in the type of filming system being used, including 1) the type of film (low-contrast or high-contrast), 2) the processing conditions (the time-temperature method of developing films should be adhered to for visualization of optimal contrast—see Chapter 9), and 3) the use of screens versus no screens. That is, because intensifying screens convert radiant energy to visible light, contrast is increased with screens; whereas without screens (direct exposure), contrast is affected mostly by the natural difference in tissue thickness.

As previously stated, contrast enhances information by making the detail of structures appropriately visible in the image. Without appropriate levels of subject contrast being visualized in the radiographic image, it would be difficult to differentiate human structures and diseases with discernible accuracy.

It was stated earlier, under the discussion on mAs, that the overall amount of density or blackness seen in the radiographic image is controlled by the quantity of mAs used and that the degree of density is proportionate to the mAs (double the mAs, double the density). By comparison, contrast is controlled by kVp and has an approximate effect on the image according to the 15% rule. This rule means that if you are using 80 kVp in your technique factors (i.e., 300 mA, .30 seconds, 80 kVp) and you add 15% (12 kVp) more to the original 80, kVp is increased to 92. Such a change would double the kVp penetration effectiveness, but contrast would visibly decrease.

Increasing or decreasing the kVp by 15% has an effect equivalent to increasing or decreasing the mAs by one half. It should be noted that although kVp and mAs have an interactive effect in increasing or decreasing contrast and density respectively, they may not be interchanged to compensate for the lack of one or the other. As further explanation, note that if structures are underpenetrated due to a lack of kVp, no amount of mAs increase will improve the penetration; added mAs will only add density. Penetration of structure can best be achieved by using the appropriate amount of kVp. Conversely, if an image is underexposed and lacks density, mAs must be added; kVp would add only scattered radiation and thus cause the image to look gray and flat without clarity.

In summary, the two factors of mAs (density) and kVp (contrast) must be used so that the interactive effects are complementary to each other and not compensatory for the lack of one or the other.

Milliamperage-Seconds (mAs) and Contrast. Milliamperage-seconds (mAs) fundamentally controls the quantity of radiation; kVp fundamentally controls contrast. The two factors must not be interchanged. Too much mAs will result in increased density or blackness with an accompanying loss of visible radiographic contrast. It is equally important to note that increasing mAs generally will not improve structure penetration, which is also controlled by kVp.

Distance and Contrast (kVp). The intensity of primary and secondary radiation changes inversely proportional to the square of the distance. Any change in distance will result in a proportionate change in the amount of scattered radiation. Thus, image contrast will not be affected. The degree of density in nearby structures may be lighter or darker, but the level of contrast will be fundamentally unchanged. Additionally, the degree of structure penetration will not, for all practical purposes, be affected. Levels of kVp penetration are equally effective at any distance (e.g., 70 kVp, 80 kVp).

Other Factors and Density and Contrast.   Other factors that influence both density and contrast are beam restriction, beam filtration, and compression of tissue. Although these areas are discussed later in the chapter, they are mentioned here to facilitate easy reference.

Beam restriction or *limitation* reduces the amount of scattered radiation interacting with the body and thereby prevents excessive scatter from fogging the film with increased density and decreased contrast of the visible image.

Beam filtration (filters) is added to the radiation beam to eliminate nonuseful soft, low-energy (long wavelengths) radiation. This filtration results in hardening of the beam by allowing mostly higher energy (shorter wavelengths) to pass through unchanged. Contrast may be improved then with a decreased amount of lower-energy wavelengths.

Compression of tissue has the effect of reducing tissue thickness. In the area where tissue is compressed, therefore, contrast may be visibly reduced due to increased penetration by kVp. Density will be increased in the same area due to less absorption of radiation.

GEOMETRIC FACTORS

Density and contrast are photographic factors that refer to the properties of the visible radiographic image. Geometric factors deal with the recorded detail of the image and the accuracy with which the true edges of the anatomy may be seen. *Recorded detail*, *distortion*, and *magnification* are the geometric factors of interest.

Recorded Detail

Recorded detail is the degree of information or definition that may be seen in the anatomy or the resolution or sharpness of lines that separates one structure from another. Although motion is rarely seen in a radiographic image because of very rapid exposure-time settings on today's equipment, motion completely destroys information by blurring the visibility of the radiographic (or recorded) image. It really does not require a great deal of experience or knowledge to recognize blurring in a radiographic image. It may be compared to the blurring seen in an ordinary photograph when the subject has moved. The fastest possible exposure time therefore is the best recourse against motion and should always be used in accordance with all other factors when making any radiographic exposure.

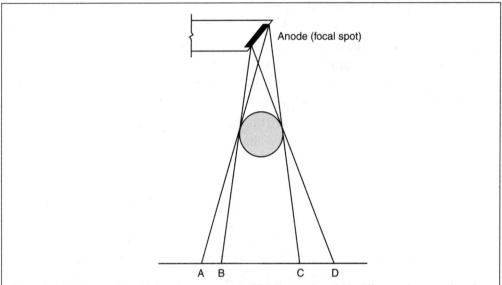

Penumbra (AB) is considerably less than penumbra (CD). Knowledge of this difference in penumbra size can be used to minimize unsharpness effects by proper positioning of the patient. In essence what is happening is that the film is seeing a smaller focal spot on the anode side as compared with the cathode side. Generally, the area of primary interest is pointed towards the anode side of the X-ray tube.

Figure 8-6 Focal spot and its relationship to subject placement *(Reprinted courtesy of Eastman Kodak Company)*

Focal-spot size (FSS), source-to-image-distance (SID), object-film distance (OFD), and intensifying screens are factors that influence the geometry of the image, and each must be designed to reduce or minimize the geometric blur. "Geometric blur," or *penumbra*, Figure 8-6, is the term used to describe the gradient unsharpness or edge enhancement of an image.

Focal-Spot Size.   The effective focal-spot size was discussed in Chapter 6. The relationship of the focal spot to geometric blur is that it is the single most important factor in recording the detail of the anatomy in the radiographic image. The smaller focal spot (produced by the smaller filament) in a dual focus tube will produce more recorded detail than the larger focal spot (filament), Figure 8-7. The rule to follow in utilizing focal-spot size is to use the smaller one whenever the exposure factors (mA, T, kVp, and SID) are set low enough to allow its use.

Source-to-Image Distance.   SID, for all practical purposes, has no effect on

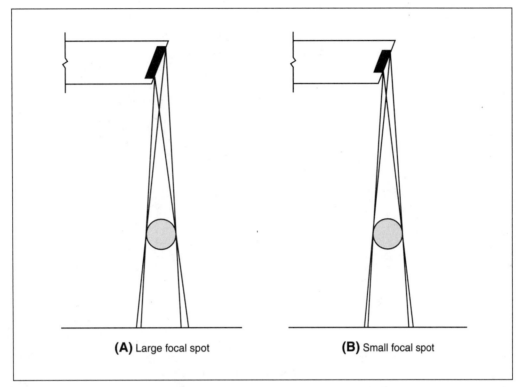

(A) Large focal spot   **(B)** Small focal spot

Figure 8-7 Penumbral shadow or edge unsharpness occurs because the focal spot on the anode is not a point source. It is comprised of many point sources, each of which projects its own object image onto the film. A) Large focal spot and its resulting penumbra; B) Small focal spot and a reduced amount of penumbra. *(Reprinted courtesy of Eastman Kodak Company)*

the penetrating power of the kVp. Changes in the SID will not affect contrast as long as the kVp remains unchanged. The rule concerning the relationship between SID and recorded detail is that a greater (increased) SID will reduce geometric blur and thus improve recorded detail. (See the penumbra reduction in Figure 8-8.) Most radiographic images are produced at a standardized forty-inch SID. (See section on distance and density, page 162.)

Object-Film Distance (OFD). OFD may also be referred to as object-image distance (OID). Either term refers to the practice/rule of placing the anatomy (object) as close to the film (in the cassette holder) as possible. This is a cardinal rule to observe in radiography because magnification occurs when the part is not close to the film. The result is an overall enlarged and fuzzy image. Although we

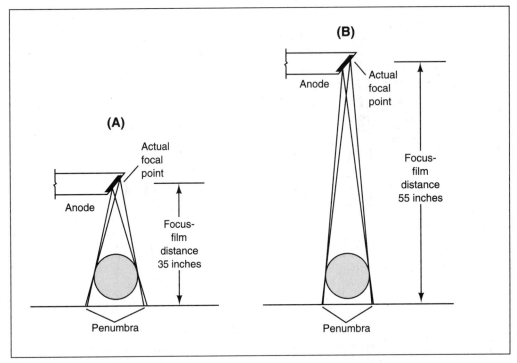

Figure 8-8   Focus-film distance is the distance between the focal spot and the film. Generally speaking, focus-film distance directly affects the degree of penumbral shadow and geometric unsharpness. Note that A has a 35-inch focus-film distance and a greater degree of penumbral shadow than B, which has a 55-inch focus-film distance. The radiographic illustrations provided graphically illustrate the difference in penumbral shadow as one goes from a short focus-film distance to a long focus-film distance. *(Reprinted courtesy of Eastman Kodak Company)*

recognize that placing the anatomy adjacent to the film surface is not always possible, minimizing the gap is important to reducing geometric blur, Figure 8-9. The rule should be to always place the part (object) adjacent to or as close as possible to the cassette surface. Magnification or size distortion may be reduced by decreasing the OFD or by increasing the SID. Most radiographs are taken at a standard SID of 40" (100 cm), which usually results in a magnification factor of approximately 1.1.

For radiographs taken at 72" (180 cm) the magnification factor is approximately 1.05. Several formulas may be used to determine the amount of image magnification. The most practical formula applies the ratio of SID to SOD (the distance from the source of the X rays to the object being examined; SOD is also referred to as FOD for focal-object distance).

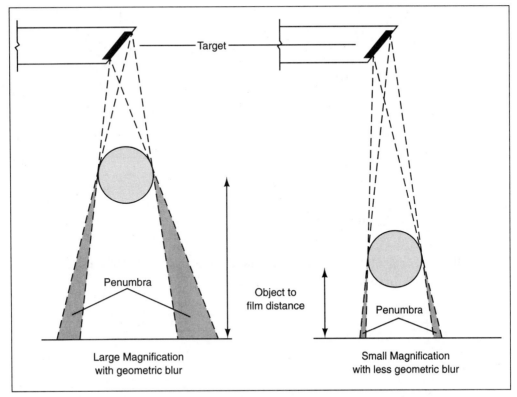

Figure 8-9 Improvement in radiographic image due to shorter object-to-film distance *(Reprinted courtesy of Eastman Kodak Company)*

$$MF = \frac{SID}{SOD}$$

$$= \frac{40}{32}$$

$$= 1.25 \text{ times}$$

These same results, however, may be arrived at in a different, but more involved, way. Determining the percentage of magnification requires certain information—that is, the size of the image width (IW) and object width (OW) must be established. While the image width may be measured from the radiograph, the object width must be determined. For example, suppose you are using a 40" SID, an 8" OFD, and a 10 centimeter (cm) image size. The following formulas may be used to determine object width and amount of magnification.

(1) $OW = \dfrac{SID}{SID - OFD}$

$ = \dfrac{40}{40 - 8} = \dfrac{40}{32}$

$\dfrac{40}{32} = \dfrac{10 \text{ cm}}{x}$

$\dfrac{40}{32} = \dfrac{10 \times 32}{40x}$

$\dfrac{320}{40} = 8 \text{ cm (OW)}$

Once the object width has been determined, the following formula may be used to be used to calculate the magnification factor.

(2) $MF = \dfrac{IW}{OW}$

$ = \dfrac{10}{8}$

$ = 1.25$

The percentage of magnification may then be calculated according to the following formula.

(3) $\%MF = \dfrac{IW - OW}{OW} \times 100$

$ = \dfrac{10 - 8}{8} \times 100$

$ = \dfrac{2}{8} \times 100$

$ = 00.25 \times 100$

$ = 25\%$

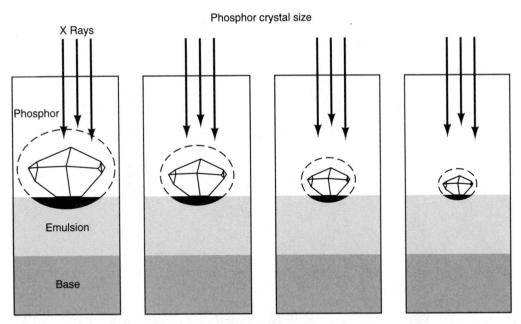

Phosphor crystal size

X Rays

Phosphor

Emulsion

Base

Figure 8-10 Various crystal sizes and the relative light spreads that occur when they are struck by incident radiation. Smaller crystal size creates less light diffusion in the radiographic image. *(Reprinted courtesy of Eastman Kodak Company)*

Intensifying Screens. Intensifying screens affect recorded detail according to the size of the phosphor crystal (see Chapter 9). Smaller crystal size will create less blurring of the image because there is less diffusion of light created by the smaller crystal, Figure 8-10. Screens are discussed in greater detail under Accessories.

Screen-Film Contact. The loss of screen-film contact is infrequent with automatic systems where no one ever touches or opens cassettes. Generally, screen-film contact is lost only in cassettes that are larger in size (14 × 17 in/ 35 × 43 cm) and when cassettes are constantly opened for loading, unloading, and cleaning. What visually appears with incomplete screen-film contact is a blurring of the image, usually in the center of the film (Figure 8-11A).

Film Resolution. Film resolution is the ability of the crystals within the film emulsion to efficiently record information. This ability is dependent on crystal size. Generally, smaller crystal size will be able to resolve and record more image information with less geometric blur than larger crystal size.

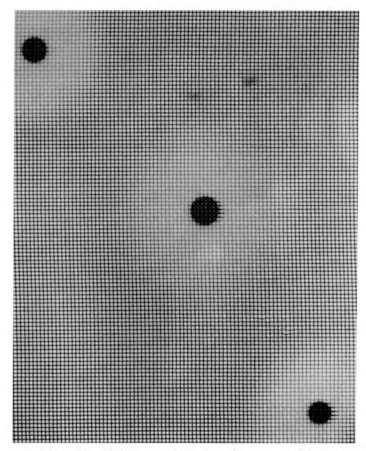

Figure 8-11A   Poor screen-film contact. These films demonstrate blurring around the areas where the coins have been placed. Poor screen-film contact appears in the area of the screens where there may be poor contact. This is more common with large 14 × 17 in. size screens than with any other size screens. *(Reprinted courtesy of Eastman Kodak Company)*

Distortion and Magnification

Distortion of the radiographic image refers to changes in size or shape of the anatomic part (as seen in real life and projected on the radiograph). Magnification (Figure 8-11B), foreshortening, and elongation (Figure 8-12) of the actual image size or shape are forms of distortion. A number of factors—object-to-film distance (OFD), distance (SID), motion, focal-spot size (FSS), and tube-to-part alignment—influence geometric factors, Figure 8-11A and B, although they do not control them (see magnification factor, page 174).

Figure 8-11B Notice the size of the coins as a result of magnification compared to the image size of the coins in Figure 8-11A. *(Reprinted courtesy of Eastman Kodak Company)*

Motion. Motion is a major factor in reducing image clarity and increasing distortion. A radiograph containing motion is referred to as a "blurred image." The blurred or fuzzy edges result in increased penumbra. Using as fast an exposure time as possible and patient-immobilization devices are the best methods to reduce image distortion caused by motion.

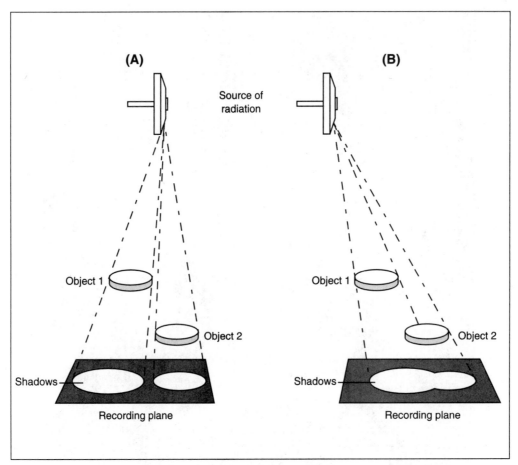

Figure 8-12 Some magnification in the radiographic image may be useful (e.g., for a finger). Distortion, however, is rarely helpful. A) No distortion in the circular objects on the recording plane (film); B) With a change in the direction (angle) of the radiation, the circular objects elongate and overlap—they appear as one object. The radiation must pass through the object perpendicularly as the object is placed parallel to the recording plane.

Tube-Part Alignment. Improper alignment of the tube or central ray to the body part or the film results in distortion. This distortion may cause the image to appear longer or shorter than its actual length. The physical shape of the anatomic part can also influence the amount of distortion. Whenever possible, to avoid shape distortion, the radiographic tube (central ray) should be perpendicular to the long axis of the part, Figure 8-13.

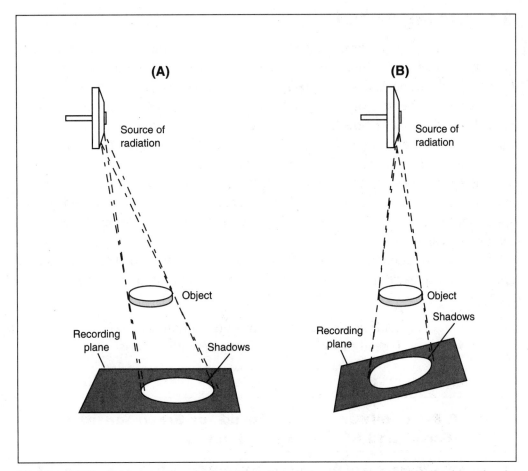

Figure 8-13 Tube-part alignment. A) Even though the source is not vertically above the circular object, it casts a circular shadow, provided the object and the recording plane are parallel; B) Distortion results when object and image-receptor plane are not parallel.

IMAGE-PRODUCTION ACCESSORIES

There are several accessory items that are very important to image production. These accessory items are generally standardized and few changes need ever be made regarding their use and application. It is important, however, to understand the purpose of and effect of these items on the image. These accessory items are: *intensifying screens*, *grids*, *beam restrictors*, *filtration*, and *processing*.

Intensifying Screens

Intensifying screens have phosphors that intensify the action of radiation. Although screens are addressed in Chapter 9, some review is appropriate here to help understand the effect of exposure with screens. Two important elements of screens are: 1) the size of the crystal and 2) thickness of the layer of the phosphor. The effect that screens have on density is related to both the crystal size and thickness of the emulsion, which determines the screen speed (response time) or amount of light produced (intensification). There are several categories of screens: detail or slow-speed screens, general purpose or medium-speed screens, and fast or high-speed screens. For convenience and ease of recognition, screen speeds have been given specific numbers by manufacturers. Some related information appears in Table 8-5.

Screen-speed factor or intensification of screens is determined as a ratio of the amount of exposure necessary without screens to the amount necessary with screens:

$$\text{Intensification factor (speed factor)} = \frac{\text{exposure without screens}}{\text{exposure with screens}}$$

TABLE 8-5 ▪ Relative Screen Speed for Green-Sensitive (Rare-Earth) and Blue-Sensitive Screens

GREEN-LIGHT-EMISSION SCREEN SPEED	RELATIVE SPEED
Detail (slow)	80–100
General purpose (medium)	250–300
Fast (high)	400–800
Ultrahigh	1200
BLUE-LIGHT-EMISSION SCREEN SPEED	**RELATIVE SPEED**
Detail (slow)	20–30
General purpose (medium)	100–200
Fast (high)	250

Note: This table lists only a few generalized screen speeds. Detailed charts showing related film types may be obtained from the appropriate screen manufacturer.

Because we are concerned with the amount of density produced in the combination of screens and film, it is more effective and efficient to think in terms of speed. That is, if one is in the process of changing screens, it is necessary to know what change in exposure factors, if any, will be required. For example, a speed factor of 100 would require 50 percent more exposure than a speed factor of 200 (see Table 8-5).

Screen speed affects density by the required exposure necessary to produce a given amount of blackness in the radiographic image. Again, using the above factors, if a general purpose screen with a rating of 200 is used and it is then decided that a detail screen with a rating of 100 is needed, an increase of 50 percent more exposure will be needed to maintain the same density with the slower detail screen. For practical purposes, however, the daily use of screens is standardized, so that exposure factors are determined according to the way in which radiographic procedures are conducted on a routine basis. Procedures may vary from extremities, chest, abdomen, pelvis, spine, and skull examinations in large radiography departments to extremities, chest, abdomen, and pelvis in smaller departments or a doctor's office.

Grids

Grids are precision instruments designed for the single purpose of absorbing scattered radiation, although some primary radiation is absorbed as well. A grid is designed to be used where density of the image is affected by the amount of scattered radiation reaching the film. This is because a greater exposure is needed for producing images of structures that measure above 12 cm in thickness, where more than 70 kVp is required. When kVp settings are increased, more scattered radiation is created. Basically, changing from no grid to the use of a grid requires four times more exposure because of scattered and primary beam absorption by lead strips in the grid, Figure 8-14. The grid works in this way: when a grid is added, it is placed under the table, between the patient and the film. The lead strips in the grid absorb divergent radiation beams scattered away from the direction of the more perpendicular primary beam. The gaps between the lead strips allow the primary beam to reach and interact with the film emulsion whereas the scattered radiation is absorbed by the lead strips. The amount of scattered radiation that is absorbed by the grid is related to *grid ratio*. Grid ratio is defined as the ratio of the height of the lead strips to the distance between the lead strips, as seen in the following diagram, Figure 8-15.

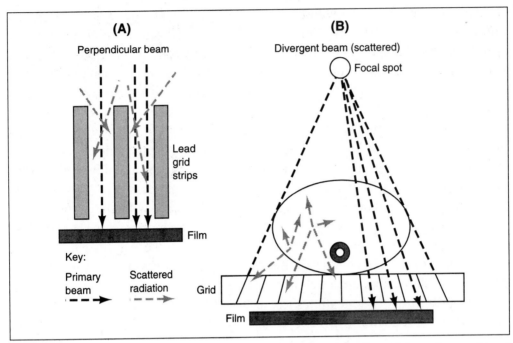

Figure 8-14   Grid cross section. A) An enlarged small portion of a grid shows how scattered radiation is absorbed by the lead strips. It also shows how perpendicular radiation from the primary beam passes between the lead strips to reach the film emulsion. B) The radiation of the radiation beam, the part being examined, the grid, and the image-recording receptor.

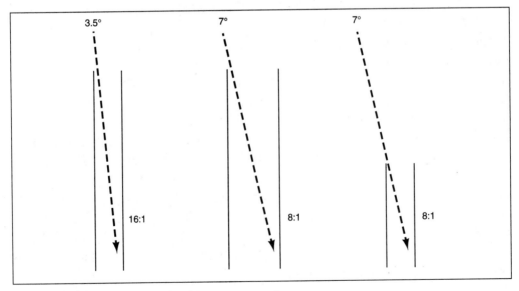

Figure 8-15   Effect of grid ratio on scatter angle

TABLE 8-6 ▪ Basic Grid Conversion Ratios for Changing from Non-Grid to Grid Technique

NON-GRID TO GRID*	WHEN mAs USE IS INCREASED	WHEN kVp USE IS INCREASED	MAXIMUM kVp FOR GRID RATIO
5:1	2 × original mAs	+ 8 kVp	80
8:1	4 × original mAs	+ 20 kVp	90–100
12:1	5 × original mAs	+ 25 kVp	110–120
16:1	6 × original mAs	+ 30 kVp	150

*Note that kVp increases may be preferable to mAs increases when technique is changed from non-grid exposure to grid exposure. An increase in mAs reduces contrast as well as increases exposure time, whereas an increase in kVp does not increase radiation dosage. Also, unless the kVp is excessive, decreasing mAs permits the penetration value of the total exposure to be retained.

As seen in the diagram, the effect of the grid lines, or its efficiency (cleanup ability), depends on the height of the lead strips and the distance between the strips (wide or narrow). The less the distance between them and greater the height, as in the 16:1 ratio, the more efficient the grid will be in pickup or removal of scattered radiation.

Approximately four times more mAs must be added when a grid is used than when a grid is not used because of absorption by the lead strips. Otherwise, there would be a loss of density that would cause the radiographic image to appear greatly underexposed. For example, if 5 mAs is used without a grid, 20 mAs must be used with a grid. (See grid conversion chart, Table 8-6.)

Beam Restriction and Filtration

These areas are discussed in Chapters 11 and 12. Their effect on density, however, can be stated relatively simply. Primary beam restriction is achieved by the use of collimators, diaphragms, and occasionally cones, Figure 8-16. The purpose of these devices is to minimize the amount of scattered radiation that reaches the film. An increase in scattered radiation reaching the film results in fog, which causes an increase in density and a resultant decrease in contrast. The primary beam should be limited or confined to the area of the structure

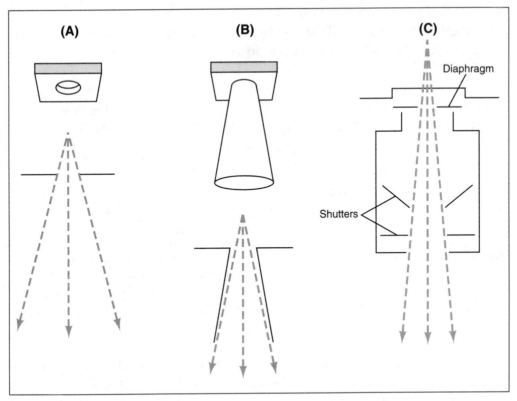

Figure 8-16 A) A sheet of lead with a hole in the center (aperture diaphragm). B) A sheet of metal or lead (diaphragm) with a cylinder cone attached. The lead is placed close to the radiation source with the cone extending down. The length and diameter of the cone determine the size of the field exposed. C) A collimator with multiple shutters. The shutters are variable by external controls, but generally are set on automatic field size. Near the tube window is a diaphragm designed to minimize off-focus radiation. The collimator is used for positive beam limitation (PBL) as required by law.

being radiographed, leaving only a narrow border within the edges of the film. The beam must at least be confined to the size of the film itself. Unnecessarily exposing large areas beyond the film edges results in added density in the radiographic image and increased dosage to the patient.

Filtration

Filtration is the process of filtering the beam of radiation through some type of material that will remove lower-energy radiation from the beam and prevent it from reaching the patient. The filter should be a type of material that will allow the more useful higher-energy radiation to pass through unchanged, but will absorb nonuseful lower-energy radiation. Aluminum is a material of choice for filters because it is less expensive than other materials and it absorbs lower-energy radiation well while allowing passage of higher-energy radiation. The aluminum is placed within the beam, either at the tube-window aperture or at the collimator opening. This is called added filtration and may measure 2.0 mm of aluminum or its equivalent. There is usually 0.5 mm of filtration within the tube itself, made up by the glass tube and its surrounding insulating oil. This is called inherent (built-in) filtration. The total minimal amount of beam filtration should be about 2.5 mm (inherent and added) of aluminum equivalent. If there were no added filtration to the radiation beam and lower-energy radiation were permitted to reach the film, the radiographic image density and patient dosage would increase. For medical radiography, patient dosage is therefore most effectively reduced with 2.5 mm of total filtration.

Processing

Three processing related elements can adversely affect film density if they are not appropriately managed. These are *safelights*, *film age*, and *chemicals*. Although these are discussed in detail in Chapter 9, a brief review is needed here. The following three requirements may be properly set by following the recommendations of the film manufacturer: 1) the safelight must have the correct color of filter for the type(s) of film used; 2) it must have the correct size (wattage) bulb; and 3) it must be placed at the correct distance from the film-loading area and processor.

Age of film is important. Film comes from the manufacturer with an expiration date. Film boxes should be stored so that the oldest film is always used prior to that more recently dated.

Processor chemicals are precisely controlled by a time-temperature processing method. Any increase in the temperature is likely to add density to the film. Also, if the chemicals are not properly replenished and become exhausted or contaminated for any reason, added chemical density will occur on the film. All of the above, if not controlled, will create fog on the film that will result in increased density.

SUMMARY

A summary of photographic factors and geometric factors appears in Table 8-7.

TABLE 8-7 ▪ Summary of Photographic and Geometric Factors

FACTORS	CONTROLLED BY	INFLUENCED/ AFFECTED BY
	Photographic Factors	
Density	mAs	SID
		Heel effect
		kVp
		Fog processing
Contrast	Kilovoltage	Filters
		Fog (all forms)
		Film processing
		Subject contrast
		Type of film
		Pathology
Secondary Radiation Fog		Size of area exposed
		Compression
		Cones
		Diaphragms
		Grids
		kVp
	Geometric Factors	
Recorded Detail		Focal-spot size
		Object-film distance
		Motion
		Screen-crystal size
		Film-screen contact
Image Size (Magnification)		Focus-film distance
		Object-film distance
Image Size (Distortion)		Alignment of tube to film
		Alignment of part to film
		Object-film distance

REVIEW QUESTIONS

1. Radiographic density is best defined as the
   a) sharpness of the radiographic image
   b) distortion of the image shape and size
   c) degree of blackness in the radiograph
   d) degree of difference between the light and dark areas

2. Radiographic contrast is best defined as the
   a) sharpness of the radiographic image
   b) distortion of the image shape and size
   c) degree of blackness in the radiograph
   d) degree of difference between the light and dark areas

3. Select the exposure setting that will result in the greatest density:

	mA	TIME	SID
a)	100	$\frac{1}{2}$ second	36"
b)	200	$\frac{1}{4}$ second	30"
c)	300	$\frac{1}{6}$ second	40"
d)	400	$\frac{1}{8}$ second	46"

4. To apply heel effect when radiographing a femur, position the thicker anatomic part beneath the
   a) cathode
   b) anode
   c) cathode or anode
   d) there is little difference

5. A sharp difference between the light and dark areas of a radiographic image is termed
   a) subject contrast
   b) long-scale contrast
   c) short-scale contrast
   d) inherent contrast

6. To change from a short-scale contrast to a long-scale contrast
   a) decrease mAs and increase kVp
   b) decrease mAs and decrease kVp
   c) increase mAs and decrease kVp
   d) increase mAs and increase kVp

7. A grid should be used when the body part being radiographed is
   a) likely to produce motion
   b) thicker than twelve centimeters
   c) subject to variations in size
   d) radiolucent

8. Which of the following technical factor sets is likely to result in the greatest amount of magnification?

	mAs	OFD	SID
a)	30	6"	36"
b)	50	5"	50"
c)	75	4"	60"
d)	100	3"	72"

9. The photographic properties of a radiograph consist of the following elements:
   a) recorded detail
   b) density and contrast
   c) magnification and distortion
   d) a and b
   e) a and c

10. The primary purpose of a grid is to reduce the effects of _____ on the image.
    a) density
    b) contrast
    c) scattered radiation
    d) all of the above

11. When any of several combinations of mA and T will produce an equivalent amount of mAs, the result is called
    a) Ohm's Law
    b) reciprocity law
    c) inverse square law
    d) none of the above

12. Heat unit (HU) capacity is determined by the following formula:
    a) $mA \times T$
    b) $mA \times kVp$
    c) $mA \times T \times kVp$
    d) $mA \times T \times kVp^2$

13. *The intensity of radiation is inversely proportional to the square of the distance* expresses the relationship between:
    a) distance and density
    b) distance and contrast
    c) distance and focal-spot size
    d) distance and radiation intensity

14. A change in SID from an original position of 40" to an increased position of 60" will change the following effect of _____.
    a) density (mA)
    b) intensity (SID)
    c) penetration (kVp)
    d) all of the above

15. The term "geometric blur" or penumbra is associated with the effects of the following factor(s):
    a) FSS
    b) SID
    c) OFD
    d) a and c
    e) a, b, c

16. When a standard 40" SID is used, the approximate amount of magnification of most radiographic images would be:
    a) 1.5
    b) 1.75
    c) 1.1
    d) 2.0

17. Primary beam filtration may be achieved by the use of a device (or devices) known as a:
    a) diaphragm
    b) cone
    c) collimator
    d) all of the above

18. The total amount of minimal beam filtration is:
    a) 2.0 mm
    b) 2.5 mm
    c) 0.5 mm
    d) none of the above

19. Which one of the grid ratios listed below is more efficient than the others?

    a) 5:1
    b) 8:1
    c) 16:1
    d) no one is more efficient than the others

20. The magnification factor is represented by the following formula:

    a) $\dfrac{\text{SID}}{\text{SOD}}$

    b) $\dfrac{\text{SID}}{\text{SID} - \text{OFD}}$

    c) $\dfrac{\text{Image Width}}{\text{Object Width}}$

    d) b only

    e) a and c

Chapter 9

Radiographic Film Processing

Chapter Outline

Objectives

Upon completion of the chapter, the student will meet the following objectives by verifying knowledge, facts, and principles presented through oral and written communication at a level deemed competent and will meet the task objectives by demonstrating the specific behavior as identified in the terminal performance objectives of the procedures.

1. Identify appropriate responses related to processing-area location, construction, and function.
2. Describe the composition of screen film and explain the function of each part.
3. Recall three characteristics of screen film.
4. Identify proper procedures for handling and storing radiographic film.
5. Outline the procedure for checking safelight illumination.
6. Explain the purpose of intensifying screens.
7. Identify the difference between calcium-tungstate and rare-earth screens.
8. Outline the procedure for proper care and cleaning of intensifying screens.
9. Discuss the basic difference between manual and automatic processing.
10. Describe the steps in film processing.
11. Explain the purpose of replenishment of processing chemicals.
12. Recognize common film artifacts and identify causative factors.
13. Demonstrate competence in each task listed. Refer to the appendix for the individual procedure/performance guides.

    TASKS (See Appendix):
    9-1 Testing Safelight Performance
    9-2 Maintaining Master Card File or Computer System
    9-3 Indexing and Filing Radiographs
    9-4 Processing Loans of Radiographs
    9-5 Loading and Unloading a Cassette
    9-6 Cleaning Intensifying Screens
    9-7 Testing Cassette for Screen-film Contact
    9-8 Processing Film by Manual Method
    9-9 Processing Film by Automatic Method

INTRODUCTION

"Film processing can make or break an otherwise perfect radiograph." This statement, common among radiographers, refers to the importance of film processing in the production of diagnostic radiographs. For proper film processing to occur, many tasks must be completed. This starts with a well-maintained darkroom environment, equipment, and supplies and ends with a fully processed diagnostic radiograph.

This chapter introduces theory about maintaining the darkroom environment, film and screen construction and proper care, film processing, and the inter-related factors involved in producing diagnostic-quality radiographs.

PROCESSING AREA CONSIDERATIONS

A processing area should offer an environment in which the necessary functions can be carried out safely and efficiently, without providing hazards that would compromise the diagnostic quality of finished radiographs. The processing area actually requires "safe" artificial light rather than total blackness. However, the processing area is still commonly called "the darkroom," and this term will be used throughout the chapter.

Location of the Darkroom

Whether they are located in an office or in a hospital, most processing areas today are automated. To save time, darkrooms are generally located near the radiographic rooms. The distance between the darkroom and radiography rooms is more important in a multi-doctor clinic or large hospital, where the patient volume may require a full-time person to perform film processing and equipment maintenance.

Darkroom ventilation should provide a constant flow of fresh air with a temperature between 60°F and 70°F. The relative humidity level should be maintained at between 40 percent and 60 percent. This prevents a buildup of chemical odors, yet allows enough air moisture to prevent static electricity that can discharge to the film and cause artifacts. A well-ventilated darkroom is also important for a healthy work environment. A film-viewing area may be adjacent to the darkroom where radiographs can be viewed, Figure 9-1. The darkroom should be large enough to provide space for loading and unloading cassettes, film storage bin, processing equipment, and related accessories.

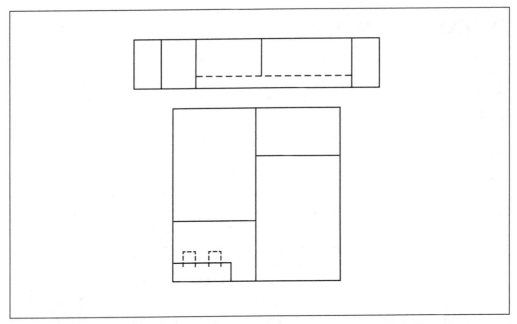

Figure 9-1 Sketch of typical darkroom arrangement with essential film viewing and processing areas identified

Walls adjacent to the radiographic rooms should be shielded with 1.6 mm (1/16 in) lead all the way to the ceiling to protect unexposed film from radiation exposure. Passboxes may be built into the walls to allow passage of cassettes between the darkroom and radiographic room. A typical passbox has two sets of doors to allow such passage between rooms and an interlock system on each set of doors to prevent accidental light exposure should both be opened at the same time, Figure 9-2. Each set of doors will have two compartments, one for exposed and one for unexposed cassettes. The ideal location for a passbox is near the film-loading bench in the darkroom.

Darkroom walls and floor should be covered with a non-porous, chemical- and stain-resistant surface (e.g., Formica®). A radiographic processing area should have a single entrance door that allows for absolute lighttight fittings. Variations on the single entrance are: 1) a maze-type entry, Figure 9-3; 2) a revolving door, Figure 9-4; and 3) an electric interlocking door system. Whatever the entrance design, the purpose is to protect radiographic film from being struck by light and/or radiation and being fogged. Processing-area lighting consists of safelight, radiographic illumination, and regular lighting.

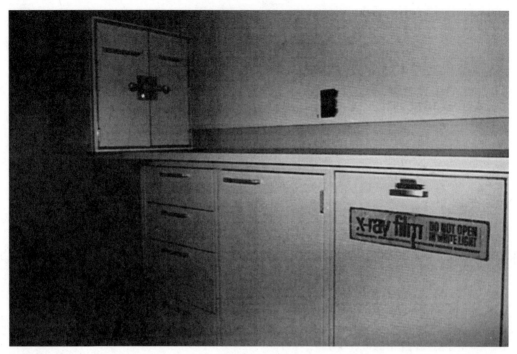

Figure 9-2 Passbox located between darkroom and radiographic room. Note double-lock doors and easy accessibility to film-loading bench. *(Reprinted courtesy of Eastman Kodak Company)*

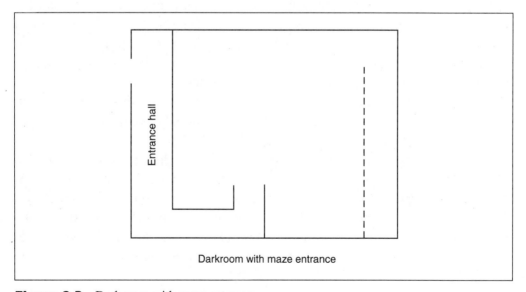

Figure 9-3 Darkroom with maze entrance

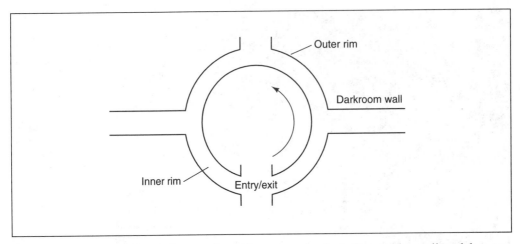

Figure 9-4 Revolving darkroom door. The outer rim is built into the wall and has two openings: one into the darkroom and one to the outside. The door's inner rim is suspended, which allows it to rotate on a central bearing. The inner rim's opening can be turned to coincide with the outer rim's openings.

RADIOGRAPHIC FILM

A radiograph is a permanent image created when ionizing radiation passes through matter and onto photographic film. The image is latent, or invisible, and will become manifest, or visible, after the film is processed. The recording medium, or radiographic film, plays a very critical role in the production of diagnostic radiographs. If the film is defective, or has been improperly stored or handled, the final diagnostic image may be less than perfect. Also, many things can happen during the film-processing stage that may detract from the diagnostic value of the radiograph. To avoid these problems, it is helpful to learn about radiographic film construction, latent image formation, types of film, and proper film handling and storage.

Radiographic film consists of two parts, the base and the emulsion, surrounded by a protective covering of gelatin called the supercoating. The base is constructed of a polyester that provides a rigid yet flexible support for the emulsion. A subcoating of adhesive covers the base and serves to bind the emulsion to the base polyester. The emulsion consists of a mixture of gelatin and silver halide crystals. Usually, 95% of the silver halide consists of silver bromide with the remainder being silver iodide.

Most radiographic film is coated on both sides and thus is called double

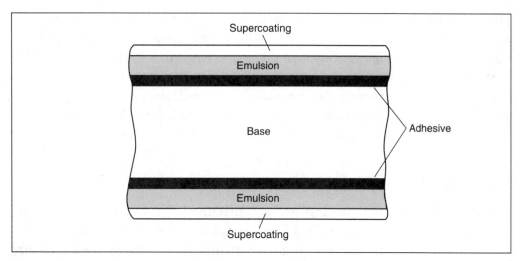

Figure 9-5   Cross section of radiographic film

emulsion film. The emulsion is the most important layer of the film because it contains the crystals that will hold the latent image formation. The gelatin in the emulsion allows for an even distribution of the silver halide crystals. Its properties allow for rapid softening in the developer solution and quick hardening in the fixer solution. Refer to Figure 9-5, a cross section of radiographic film. The emulsion reaction to ionizing radiation can be altered by the way the crystals are manufactured and their mixture. Each manufacturer of film closely guards the unique formulas that are responsible for its film characteristics. Film characteristics include speed, contrast, and resolution. Each of these areas will be included in the discussion on film types.

Latent Image Formation

As ionizing radiation exits from matter and strikes radiographic film, energy is deposited in the emulsion. The transfer of information between the radiation and film emulsion is by photoelectric interaction. Each silver halide crystal has on its surface sensitive specks of tiny particles of atomic silver and silver sulfide. When these specks are struck by ionizing radiation, ionization of the silver halide crystals results in charged silver ions and negatively charged bromine ions, expressed as:

$$AgBr + X \text{ rays} \rightarrow Ag^+ + Br^-$$

These sensitized specks will react to the developer chemicals during film processing. Silver halide crystals that have been ionized (irradiated) will be changed into black grains through the development process. Silver halide crystals that have not been ionized will remain in crystal form and will not be changed during the development stage of film processing. These unexposed, undeveloped silver halide crystals will react to the fixer chemicals and will be released from the emulsion in the fixation step of processing and recovered through a silver-recovery chamber.

Types of X-ray Film

Many different types of film are manufactured for medical radiography. This variety reflects the diversity of radiographic procedures requiring special application film, such as those used in mammography, cardiography, dental radiography, and so forth. Limited radiographers will generally use only the two common types of X-ray films, screen-type film and direct exposure film (often called nonscreen film). The major differences between the two types of film are the thickness of the film emulsion and its response to both X ray and light emitted from the intensifying screen.

Direct exposure film responds best to X-ray. Direct exposure film is rarely used today because (1) its increased emulsion-silver content makes it more costly and (2) it requires a much higher X-ray exposure. *Because direct exposure film requires an increase in X-ray exposure, its use does not justify the increase in radiation exposure to the patient.* By using screen-type film, the radiation exposure to the patient can be reduced. This is possible because screen film (sensitive to light) is used with intensifying screens that emit light during the X-ray exposure, thereby allowing a reduction in the X-ray exposure.

Screen film has three characteristics that are routinely considered: contrast (high or low), speed (sensitivity), and light absorption. Each film manufacturer produces screen film with a certain level of contrast. This level may be high-contrast, which produces a very black-and-white shaded image, or low-contrast, which produces a gray shaded image. The film contrast of a particular brand of film is directly related to the latitude or range of exposure factors (mA, time, kVp) that will produce an acceptable image. Usually film manufacturers provide two or more latitudes, referred to as medium- or high-contrast film. The physician who is responsible for interpreting the radiographic image may wish to select the level of film contrast to be used for most radiographic procedures.

Screen film is also available in different speeds or sensitivity. The speed of a screen film refers to how fast the silver halide crystals in the emulsion respond to the light emitted from the intensifying screens. High-speed (fast) screen film contains a thick emulsion, large crystals, or a higher concentration of crystals in the emulsion. Visibility of anatomic detail on the finished radiograph may be decreased with the use of high-speed screen film. An advantage, however, of this type of film is the faster exposure times can be used. Film-speed and contrast-level selection should be a collective effort of the radiographer and physician.

Spectral absorption, commonly called spectral matching, refers to the use of film whose sensitivity is correctly matched to the light spectrum emitted from the intensifying screen. Calcium-tungstate intensifying screens emit blue and blue-violet light and should be matched to silver halide emulsion film or blue-sensitive film. Rare-earth intensifying screens should be matched to screen film that is sensitive to green light. However, they may also be compatible with blue-sensitive film. Correct spectral matching is also referred to as film-screen combination or spectral system. Selecting the correct combination is very important because if the match is incorrect, the film will not respond properly and the patient may receive more radiation than necessary because incorrect exposure may result in a repeat radiograph.

Because X-ray film is sensitive to light, the lamps or safelights used in the darkroom must meet certain requirements. Darkroom lamps are used to provide a minimum of light to allow the operator some illumination. Because exposed screen film is approximately eight times more sensitive to light than unexposed film, safelights must have their light filtered. For blue-sensitive film, an amber (Wratten 6-B) light generally is used. An amber filter will only allow light having wavelengths longer than 550 mm, or beyond the spectral response of blue-sensitive film, to be emitted. A reddish brown filter is used with green-sensitive film and can also be used with blue-sensitive film. Safelights should be installed at least three feet from the area where the film will be handled and processed. Light bulb wattage in the safelight should not exceed the manufacturer's recommendations for the specific type filter.

Safelights are designed for either indirect ceiling illumination or direct illumination. One way to determine whether a safelight is actually safe is to check the safelight illumination, evaluate the results, and take necessary action if an unsafe condition exists. Remember that safelight illumination as well as light leaks into the darkroom area and can cause fog or an undesirable film darkening that decreases the diagnostic value of the radiograph. It is important to periodically check the safelight filter for cracks and light-leaks in the lamp (filter) housing. Exercise 9-1 in the Appendix will help you practice how to test safelight performance.

Film Identification

Patient identification, date, right or left marker, and other data must be (legally) permanently marked on a radiograph. Two common methods of identification are: (1) attaching lead markers to the cassette before the exposure is made, Figure 9-6A and (2) a photographic transfer of data, Figure 9-6B. Generally, both

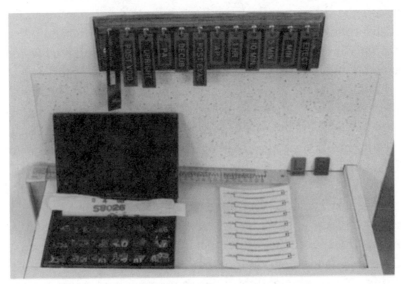

Figure 9-6A Film identification markers

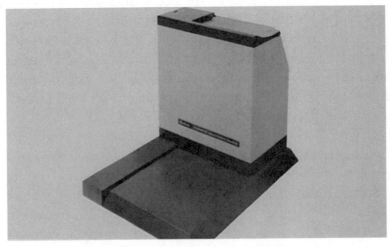

Figure 9-6B Photographic transfer of patient information to the radiograph *(Reprinted courtesy of Eastman Kodak Company)*

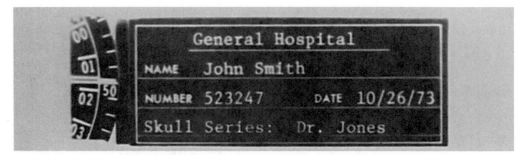

Figure 9-7 Identification information as it appears on radiograph *(Reprinted courtesy of Eastman Kodak Company)*

methods are used. The lead marker contains the patient's identification number, date, a right or left letter, and the doctor or facility name. The photographic marker usually contains more detailed data such as the patient's address, sex, age, religion, insurance identification, etc., Figure 9-7.

In the photographic method of identification, a card containing the patient data is inserted into a camera device. With the white lights off, the exposed radiograph is placed in the camera window, and a very quick light exposure is made, thereby transferring the patient data to the film, Figure 9-8. Cassettes used with this

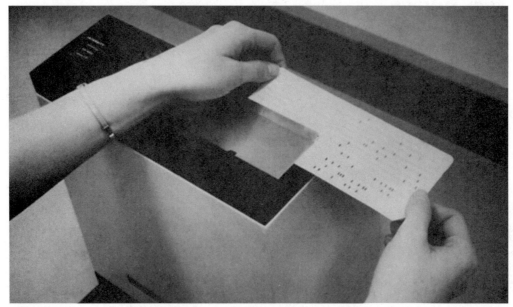

Figure 9-8 Inserting identification card into top of camera *(Reprinted courtesy of Eastman Kodak Company)*

method of identification must have a lead blocker that protects the area of the film that will later be imprinted with patient data. See also Chapter 3, page 55, Film Labeling/Identification.

RADIOGRAPHIC-FILM STORAGE AND HANDLING

Radiographic film is sensitive to X rays, heat, light, chemical fumes, moisture, pressure, and any kind of rough handling, i.e., bending, scratching, crimping, etc. Radiographic film must be properly stored and carefully handled to ensure that damage does not occur.

Film Packaging

Radiographic film is packaged in a moisture-free, sealed bag with cardboard supports. The bag is packaged in a heavy duty plastic bag within a sealed cardboard shipping carton. The outside of the carton indicates the type of film, quantity, and expiration date. Film is available in quantities of twenty-five, fifty, and one hundred sheets per carton. Individually wrapped sheets of film can also be purchased; such film is called interleaved or prewrapped film.

Film Storage

Radiographic film should be stored in a cool, dry place. The temperature of the storage area has a direct influence on the length of time unexposed film can be maintained and used (refer to Table 9-1). The best temperature for film storage is

TABLE 9-1 ▪ Film Storage Temperature/Time Length Usable Relationships	
MAINTAINED STORAGE TEMPERATURE	APPROXIMATE LENGTH OF TIME FILM STAYS USABLE
90–100°F	2–3 days
70°F	2 months
60°F	6 months
50°F	1 year

between 60°F and 70°F and 40% and 60% relative humidity. Stored film should also be protected from x-radiation, fumes, chemicals, and any gas-producing substance. Film boxes should never be subjected to excessive pressure. To avoid pressure marks, warping, and bending, boxes of unexposed film should always be stored upright.

Stored film should be used prior to the expiration date. Stored film boxes should be rotated as new shipments arrive. Rotate the stock so that film with the most recent expiration date is always used first. This avoids having to discard expired film and saves money in film expense.

Once a film box is opened, a film bin, Figure 9-9, provides ideal storage. A film bin has separate compartments to hold different film sizes and is usually installed beneath the film loading area. Film bins may be electrically connected to the overhead lights. In this case, the lights will not turn on if the film bin drawer is open. Also, the darkroom entrance door may be electrically connected to the film bin to prevent accidental light exposure to the film should the door be opened while the bin is open.

Film fog is defined as an undesirable increase in the density of the emulsion, either before or after radiation exposure. The additional film density or fog decreases the quality of the radiographic image by reducing the visibility of the diagnostic information. Light is only one of several causes of fog. Refer to Table 9-2 for a brief listing of the causes of fog.

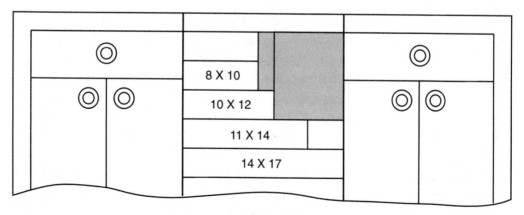

Figure 9-9 Film bin. A film bin is generally installed in existing counter space.

TABLE 9-2 ▪ Causes of Film Fog

SOURCE	PRECAUTION TO AVOID
Chemical Fumes	Certain chemical fumes will cause the emulsion to become fogged. Do not store films in an area that contains chemical fumes and is poorly ventilated.
Temperature and Humidity	Store films in an area with 40%–50% relative humidity and constant temperature range between 60–70°F.
Radiation	Film must be stored in an area where it is protected from radiation. Stored film must be protected from primary and secondary scatter radiation.
Pressure	Store film boxes on edge, never stack them. Avoid dropping film boxes.
Age	Use film before the expiration date indicated on the film box. Rotate stock.

Film Handling

X-ray film must be handled carefully to avoid extraneous marks and images on the radiograph; such marks or images are called artifacts. An artifact can also be defined as an area of increased or decreased film darkening or density. Handle film carefully, avoiding creasing or bending and rapid movement of the film, which can cause static electric discharges to be conveyed to the film, Figure 9-10. Proper loading and unloading of cassettes and direct-exposure film envelopes are essential.

When films are carelessly handled by an individual loading and unloading cassettes, the films may be bent. This damages the emulsion and results in artifacts called crescent or crinkle marks, semicircular in shape. A white crescent-shaped mark results from bending the film before exposure. A black crescent-shaped mark is caused from bending the film after it has been exposed.

Film should also always be handled with clean, oil-free, and dry hands. Film-handling errors are one cause of film artifacts. For further information on film artifacts, refer to the "film processing" section of this chapter.

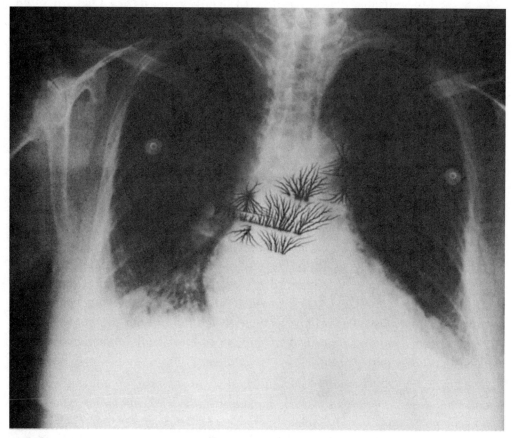

Figure 9-10 Artifacts resulting from static electric discharges to the film

Maintaining Radiographic Film

Processed radiographs are a permanent, legal patient record and should be stored at 60° to 70°F temperature and 40–50% relative humidity. The storage area should be free of chemical fumes, moisture, and excessive changes in temperature or humidity.

Each facility establishes a particular protocol for film filing and retrieval. It is important that the system provide quick access to the records as needed. Film filing folders should be made of materials that do not contain chemicals that can react with the stored radiographs. There are many ways to file and maintain radiographs. Exercises 9-2 and 9-3 in the Appendix illustrate two procedures that are among many possible methods in current use today.

Each facility will also determine how to handle requests for loans of radiographs. One example would include information on who may request films, whether a written request is required, and if all or only the most recent radiographs are provided. Rather than loan original radiographs, a facility may provide duplicates at a nominal charge. Duplication of radiographs allows the facility to maintain a complete record, yet share the information with others providing medical care to the same patient. Exercise 9-4 in the Appendix outlines a suggested protocol for loaning radiographs.

INTENSIFYING SCREENS

In 1895, German physicist Wilhelm Conrad Roentgen was operating a vacuum tube when he noticed a glow coming from a cardboard coated with a chemical, barium platinocyanide. The vacuum tube was covered so that no light escaped, yet the glow or fluorescence from the cardboard seemed to intensify when it was moved closer to the tube. Roentgen called his discovery "x-radiation" and began to investigate its properties further. In 1901, Roentgen won the first Nobel prize in physics for his discovery. His investigation led not only to the discovery and application of x-radiation but also to the use of chemically coated fluorescent screens in radiography.

> The very thing that makes x-rays useful—their penetrating power—also makes them difficult to record. For example, of the x-ray intensity in the primary beam emerging from the patient, only about 1 or 2 percent is absorbed by a sheet of x-ray film and 98 percent or more is wasted. Early in the history of x-rays, the need to use more of this wasted x-ray energy was recognized. This led to the coating of photosensitive emulsion on both sides of the x-ray plate, doubling the absorption of the single-coated material. It also led to the introduction of fluorescent intensifying screens.[1]

Since less than 2% of the X rays produced are absorbed by the film emulsion, the light emitted by the intensifying screens increases the effect on the emulsion, thereby allowing a decrease in X-ray exposure to the patient. In the last decade, the most dramatic reductions in radiation exposure to patients have resulted from the introduction of intensifying screens that have rare-earth phosphors capable of emitting even greater amounts of light.

Intensifying screens look like thin sheets of plastic. They are available in sizes corresponding to film sizes. Screens are mounted inside cassettes. Screens, like radiographic film, consist of layers, each having a specific purpose. Most intensifying screens have four layers: protective coating, phosphor, reflective layer, and base, Figure 9-11.

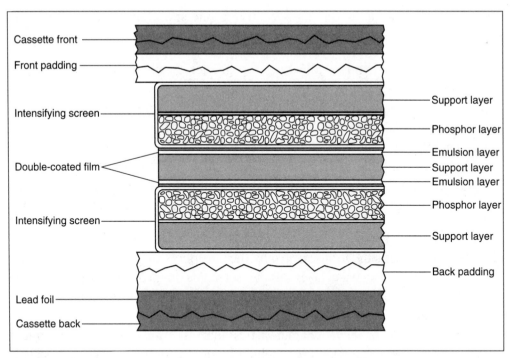

Figure 9-11 Loaded cassette with the four layers identified *(Reprinted courtesy of Eastman Kodak Company)*

The protective coating is the outermost layer of the screen and is closest to the film. This coating is transparent and serves to reduce abrasion that would damage the screen surface. It also reduces the accumulation of static electricity. This protective surface may be cleaned without causing damage to the active fluorescent phosphor.

The phosphor, or active layer, is responsible for emitting light when struck by X rays. Another way of expressing this phenomenon is to say that the phosphor is responsible for converting the energy of the X-ray beam into visible light. Phosphors used in screens may be crystalline calcium tungstate, zinc sulfide, barium lead sulfate, or the rare-earths gadolinium, lanthanum, and yttrium. Today, however, calcium tungstate or the rare earths are most commonly in use. Although rare-earth phosphor screens are more costly, they are the phosphor most often used. The major advantage of rare-earth screens over conventional calcium-tungstate screens is speed. Since rare-earth screens are faster, they require less X-ray exposure to the patient. Differences in intensifying screens result from the differences in the phosphor composition, concentration, and crystal size.

For a phosphor to be used in an intensifying screen, it must have the following properties:

1. A high atomic number allowing for greater X-ray interaction with the phosphor
2. A high *conversion efficiency*, or the ability to emit a great amount of light
3. *Spectral matching*, meaning that the light emitted is of a wavelength (color) to match the sensitivity of the X-ray film
4. Should not continue to flow or emit light after the X-ray interaction stops. *Phosphorescence* is the continued emission of light by the phosphor after the exposure has ended. This is often referred to as screen afterglow or screen lag.

The reflective layer of the screen is between the phosphor and the base. The reflective layer keeps the light emitted by the phosphors directed toward the film.

The purpose of the base layer of the screen is to provide support for the phosphor layer. It consists of a tough polyester that is chemically inert, flexible, and resists damage from the radiation.

Intensifying screens have characteristics that are important to the limited radiographer. These characteristics include intensification factor (screen speed) and resolution. The intensification factor measures the speed of the screen. Screen speed is defined simply as the screen's ability to produce density with a given exposure to X rays. There are three major speed categories of calcium-tungstate screens: medium speed, high speed, and fine detail (slow) speed. Rare-earth screens can be up to twelve hundred times faster than the categories listed for calcium-tungstate screens. Generally, these categories are described by comparing one against the others. Screen speed cannot be accurately measured, so in most discussions, the speeds will be compared in relation to their use and results.

The higher the speed of the screen, the more density will be produced at a given exposure. Use of high-speed screens reduces radiation exposure to the patient. This is possible because a greater intensification (more light) is produced by the high-speed screen, therefore, less exposure is needed to produce an image.

Although medium- and fine-detail-speed screens are available, most limited radiographers will use high-speed screens or rare-earth screens. Medium- and fine-detail-speed screens are used for specialty radiography when increased visibility of anatomic detail is desired. However, the patient may receive more radiation exposure with medium- and fine-detail-speed screens than with fast-speed screens or rare-earth screens.

Resolution is another important characteristic of intensifying screens. It is defined as the ability of a system to consistently produce an image of an object. To demonstrate resolution, one might look through a camera lens. If the object being viewed is out of focus, it has poor resolution. A rule of thumb to remember about screen resolution is that those conditions that increase the intensification factor reduce resolution. This means that high-speed screens with their large-size phosphor crystals will have a lower resolution than fine detail screens. Resolution increases as the phosphor crystals become smaller and the phosphor layer thinner. As previously mentioned, one can increase resolution with fine detail screens; however, the patient radiation exposure increases because these screens require more exposure than do fast-speed or rare-earth screens.

The choice of a film-screen combination, or film-imaging system, can significantly affect the patient's radiation exposure and the diagnostic quality of the radiation. A rule to follow regarding the selection of film and screens is to use the type and speed of film for the particular screen (e.g., high-speed film with a high-speed intensifying screen).

Direct Exposure or Cassette

Two types of film holders are used for radiography examinations: a direct exposure holder or a cassette that contains intensifying screens. Both film-holding devices will be discussed; however, direct exposure film holders are rarely used because of the increase in exposure required. Because cassettes contain a pair of intensifying screens that light up when struck by radiation, the patient's exposure dose is less than is required by a direct exposure holder containing no intensifying screens.

A direct exposure film holder, commonly called a "cardboard," is a lightproof envelope. Direct exposure (nonscreen) film is used with this type of film holder. These holders have a radiographic tube side that must face the tube during the exposure and a back side lined with lead foil to prevent scatter radiation from striking the film. Direct film holders are used for radiography of thin body parts measuring less than twelve centimeters. The advantage of direct exposure is that it provides good resolution or detail of the image. This results from the direct information transfer to the film as compared to the intensification factor of intensifying screens where some detail is lost as a result of the delay in light emitted by the crystal phosphors. *Today, however, the potential benefit of direct exposure cannot be justified because of the increase in radiation exposure required as compared to using a cassette.*

A cassette is a rigid holder containing intensifying screens. The front surface, or tube side, is made of thin, yet sturdy, plastic. The back of the cassette provides some type of spring closure device to maintain an even pressure on the film when the holder is closed. Attached to the inside are the front and back intensifying screens. A compression material such as felt is installed between each screen and the cassette cover. This material serves to further provide a good film-screen contact when the cassette is closed. Proper film loading and unloading is important in maintaining the surface of the screen as well as the condition of the film. Exercise 9-5 in the Appendix will help you learn how to properly load and unload film from a cassette.

The outside of a cassette may be cleaned with a disinfectant as frequently as necessary. The intensifying screens, however, require regular inspection and cleaning. Care must be taken to keep the screens dry and to avoid stains and scratches that may cause permanent damage. Common types of soiling are from blood, lipstick, hair dressing, and processing solutions. Foreign objects, such as small pieces of paper, hair, etc., can also find their way into a cassette. Static electricity can cause dust particles to be attracted to the screen. Many commercial screen-cleaning solutions include an antistatic compound to reduce static electricity.

Always remember the important contribution of light energy that intensifying screens make to the formation of the latent image. With this in mind, it is easy to understand that any stain, soil, or matter on the screen surface can interfere with the amount of light reaching the film. An object or stain on a screen surface will appear as an unwanted shadow or artifact on the finished radiograph.

Keeping cassettes closed and properly stored away from moisture will help to avoid damage to the intensifying screens. This also protects the screen's phosphors from light, which can weaken the chemical fluorescence of the phosphor.

A cassette that is closed and latched is assumed to be loaded with unexposed film. If, at any time, a cassette must be closed and latched without film, identify it with a note stating that it is unloaded. This precaution will help to avoid a repeat examination and unnecessary radiation exposure to a patient.

Good darkroom housekeeping to keep the darkroom and film-loading areas clean is essential. Screens should be cleaned according to the manufacturer's instructions, which often recommend a specific commercial cleaning solution. Also, cleaning solutions for calcium-tungstate screens may not be suitable for rare-earth screens because of optical residue that can interfere with the light emission. The frequency at which intensifying screens are cleaned depends upon a number of factors: manufacturer's suggested cleaning schedule, amount of use the screens receive, and overall cleanliness of the darkroom environment and operator. Exercise 9-6 in the Appendix is a sample procedure for cleaning intensifying screens.

Screen-Film Contact

Intensifying screens must be in direct contact with the film across its entire surface. Poor screen-film contact results in a severe loss of recorded detail and a slight decrease in density on the finished radiograph. The compression material (such as felt) and metal backings on the cassette are responsible for proper screen-film contact, Figure 9-12. As a result of constant use or abuse, the compression material, spring latches, or backing may become warped. When this happens, even pressure is not exerted on the screens, which causes poor screen-film contact. Other factors that can contribute to poor screen-film contact are: (1) air trapped between screen and film, (2) foreign matter on the screen surface, and (3) improperly mounted screens. The loss of screen-film contact may be gradual, and for this reason, the contact should be checked on a regular basis. Exercise 9-7 in the Appendix provides practice in checking for poor screen-film contact.

FILM PROCESSING

Chemical processing changes the latent image held in the film emulsion into a manifest image. In the early days of radiography, film processing was done manually, by moving the film from the developer to the fixer tank by hand. Drying of the radiograph was accomplished by the clothesline method of air drying. Needless to say, manual processing was not always a precise procedure and often did not allow for consistent processing results. Today, most medical facilities have automatic film processors; however, a brief section will be included on manual processing because many small medical clinics may still use this method. The basic steps of film processing are similar for automatic and manual processing: development, fixation, wash, and drying processes. The chemicals used in each method are similar, except that the strength concentration is higher for automatic processor chemistry. Also, of course, automatic processing involves higher solution temperatures and shorter processing times.

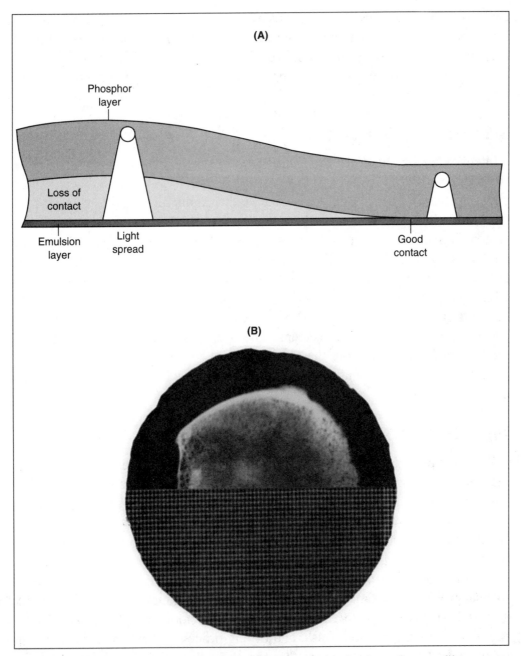

Figure 9-12 Test for screen-film contact. A) Diagram showing loss of screen-film contact; B) Radiograph showing effect of poor screen-film contact. *(Reprinted courtesy of Eastman Kodak Company)*

Overview of Film-Processing Steps

Each step will be discussed in greater detail, but it helps to form a mental image of the steps required to process a radiograph. After the cassette is unloaded in the darkroom, the exposed film is ready to be developed. The developer is responsible for converting the exposed silver halide crystals into metallic silver. The fixer actually performs two important functions: it removes the unexposed and undeveloped silver halide crystals from the emulsion and hardens the soft gelatin. The washing process removes fixer solution from the film emulsion. Drying the radiograph prepares it for viewing and later storage.

Processing Solutions

Tables 9-3 and 9-4 list the chemical ingredients of the developer and fixer.

Preparation of Solutions

Preparation of solutions is a very important step in processing. Chemical solutions should be prepared according to the manufacturer's directions and safety specifications. The following general precautions are reprinted from the *Fundamentals of Radiography*, 12th edition.[2]

General Precautions. It is extremely important to avoid chemical contamination of processing solutions because minute quantities of impurities can produce undesirable effects. Therefore:

1. Clean tanks and covers thoroughly before starting to mix fresh solutions.
2. Be careful not to splash ingredients of one solution into another. For example, small amounts of fixer can significantly change developer behavior. Be sure to use splash guards and drip trays when removing or installing processor racks because solutions can drip and contaminate other chemical tanks.
3. Use mixing and storage containers made of corrosion-resistant materials (enamel, hard-glazed earthenware, polyethylene, polypropylene, glass, hard rubber, ANSI Type 316 stainless steel with 2–3% molybdenum). Never use containers made of reactive materials such as tin, copper, zinc, aluminum, or galvanized iron.
4. Do not use tanks or other containers that have been soldered because the reaction of the solution with the solder metals causes chemical fog on film.

TABLE 9-3 ▪ Developer Chemistry

SOLVENT	Water	Dissolves the developer chemicals and causes gelatin in film emulsion to swell
DEVELOPING AGENTS	Phenidone (automatic processing) Elon and hydroquinone (manual processing)	Converts exposed silver halide crystals into metallic silver
ACCELERATORS	Sodium or potassium hydroxide	An alkali added to the developer to increase the chemical activity
PRESERVATIVES	Sodium sulfite	Prevents oxidation
RESTRAINERS	Potassium bromide Potassium iodide	Controls activity of reducing agents and prevents chemical fog
HARDENER	Glutaraldehyde	**ONLY** used for automatic processing; controls swelling of the emulsion

TABLE 9-4 ▪ Fixer Chemistry

SOLVENT	Water	Dissolves the fixer chemicals
CLEARING AND FIXING AGENTS	Ammonium thiosulfate (Hypo)	Dissolves and removes undeveloped silver halide crystals and changes the unexposed areas of the film from milky to clear and translucent
PRESERVATIVES	Sodium sulfite	Prevents decomposition of the clearing agents
HARDENER	Aluminum chloride or Potassium alum	Shrinks and hardens the emulsion
ACIDIFIER	Acetic acid	Provides an acid pH and neutralizes the alkaline developer
BUFFER		Chemicals added to fixing solution to stabilize and balance the acid-alkaline pH of the solutions

5. Cover solution tanks when not in use to keep out dirt and reduce the rate of oxidation and evaporation. The tank cover can either fit over the top or float on the solution.

6. Use two stirring paddles or plungers—one for the developer and one for the fixer. Identify and keep them separate for each solution. After use, wash them in warm water and hang them up to dry.

7. Be very careful if mercury thermometers are used for measuring solution temperatures. If such a thermometer is broken, the mercury is hazardous because of its toxicity. Also, mercury can produce a high fog level on film.

8. Finally, adjust the temperature of the water in which the chemicals are to be dissolved as recommended on package labels.[3]

Processing chemicals are available in dry and liquid form. It is important to follow the manufacturer's directions for mixing chemicals. Some general precautions include:

1. Dry chemicals should be mixed away from stored film.
2. Liquid chemicals should be mixed with water of the same temperature.
3. All chemicals should be thoroughly stirred while mixing.
4. Follow recommended safety precautions regarding inhaling chemical vapors or dry particles and eye and skin contact when using processing chemicals.

As in any chemical reaction, optimum conditions of time, temperature, and strength of solutions are critical to the process. It is best to purchase processing chemicals that are compatible to the film so that the manufacturer's recommendations regarding ideal conditions can be followed to the letter. Like film-screen combinations, it is best to have a compatible film-processing system.

Processing Steps

The four steps to be considered in film processing are developing, fixing, washing, and drying. The developer is an alkaline solution that converts exposed silver halide crystals to metallic silver by a chemical reaction. This reaction is often called a reduction process because the silver ion is said to be reduced to metallic silver.

The developer contains water, which is a solvent for the other chemicals and softens the film's emulsion. Hydroquinone is the main ingredient of developer solution with phenidone and Metol® as secondary agents. Hydroquinone and elon are combined for manual processing and hydroquinone and phenidone for rapid processing. These chemicals, when combined, have many electrons that are easily released to neutralize the positive silver ions in the film emulsion. Hydroquinone is responsible for bringing out the blackest shades on the radiograph, whereas phenidone influences the gray shades. Glutaraldehyde (hardener) is included in the developer for automatic processing. It is added to control emulsion swelling.

Unexposed silver halide crystals have a positive electrostatic charge whereas exposed silver halide crystals have a negative electrostatic charge. Because the electrostatic charge of the developer chemicals is negative, the chemicals cannot penetrate the silver halide crystal *except* in the region of exposure or where there are sensitized specks. In these areas, the developer chemicals penetrate through to the exposed specks and reduce the silver ions to atomic silver, Figures 9-13 and 9-14. Unexposed silver halide crystals are not changed or affected by the developer solution.

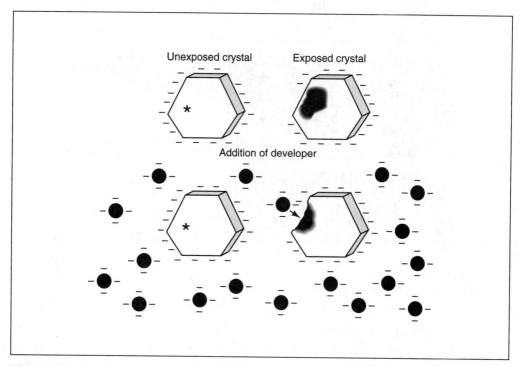

Figure 9-13 Development amplifies the latent image. Only crystals that contain a latent image are reduced to metallic silver by the addition of developer.

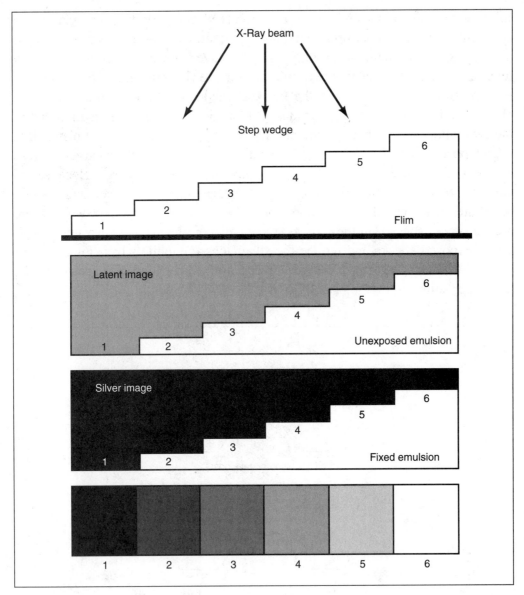

Figure 9-14   Latent image process

Other ingredients in the developer consist of an activator (such as sodium carbonate), a preservative, and restrainer. The preservative sodium sulfite serves to retard the activity of the reducing agents, thereby decreasing oxidation. Oxidation is undesirable because the chemicals' activity level declines when combined with oxygen. Potassium bromide, a restrainer, limits the action of the developer chemicals to the reduction of only the exposed silver halide crystals. Without proper balance provided by the restrainer, the unexposed silver halide crystals would be attacked. This ingredient is not required when mixing replenishment chemicals because bromide is redeposited into the solution as each film is developed. Because the potassium bromide is used when mixing the initial developer solution, it is commonly called "starting solution" or "starter."

Replenishment of chemicals is very important in providing diagnostic-quality radiographs. Replenishment is used to restore both developer and fixer chemicals to their original strength. As films are processed, they retain a certain amount of chemicals and this depletes the solution level and the chemical strength. In automatic film processing, a pump replenishes the chemicals each time a film is processed; in manual film processing, the amount and rate of replenisher chemical must be performed by the radiographer. In manual processing, replenishment is usually done daily and is based upon the number and size of the films processed.

The fixer is an acidic solution that clears or removes unexposed silver halide crystals from the film emulsion. It also hardens and fixes the film so that it can be maintained as a permanent record. The fixer, like the developer, contains water as a solvent, which serves as a base for the other chemicals. Acetic acid allows the use of potassium alum as a hardening agent but also neutralizes any alkaline developer solution remaining on the film. The clearing agent ammonium thiosulfate (hypo) removes unexposed and undeveloped silver halide crystals from the emulsion. Hardening agents, either aluminum chloride or potassium alum, control the swelling of the emulsion and help to shrink it. Sodium sulfite is included as a chemical preservative to reduce oxidation.

A film must be properly washed to remove processing chemicals. In manual processing, films must be washed in continuously circulating fresh water. Automatic processors accomplish this by a constant inflow of water.

Automatic film processors have a system that produces a dry film. In the manual system, films may be either air dried on racks or placed in a film dryer. Films should be thoroughly dry before being filed and stored. Wet or damp radiographs may stick together, rendering them useless for future reference.

Manual-Processing Considerations

The maintenance of chemical strength, tank level, and temperature are the most important considerations in manual processing. The temperature of the chemicals is maintained by water circulating around the inner tanks and by the room temperature. In the manual method, processing time is closely related to temperature and chemical strength. Manufacturers usually recommend developing at 68°F for five minutes. Rapid manual-processing chemicals are available that allow development times of less than five minutes. Manual-processing tanks must be kept covered when not in use to prevent oxidation. Figure 9-15 illustrates the conventional arrangement of a small tank unit and Figure 9-16 a single wash compartment.

The steps in manual processing and a suggested time temperature chart, Figures 9-17 and 9-18, are provided by the Eastman Kodak Company. Exercise 9-8 in the Appendix provides guidelines for manually processing film.

Automatic Film Processing

Automatic film processing, introduced in the late 1950s, has several advantages over manual processing. It is a clean and dry process; the operator does not have contact with the processing chemicals. Automatic processing is definitely faster.

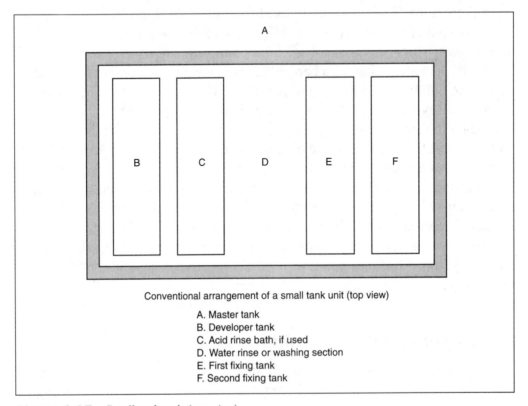

Conventional arrangement of a small tank unit (top view)

A. Master tank
B. Developer tank
C. Acid rinse bath, if used
D. Water rinse or washing section
E. First fixing tank
F. Second fixing tank

Figure 9-15   Small tank unit (*top view*)

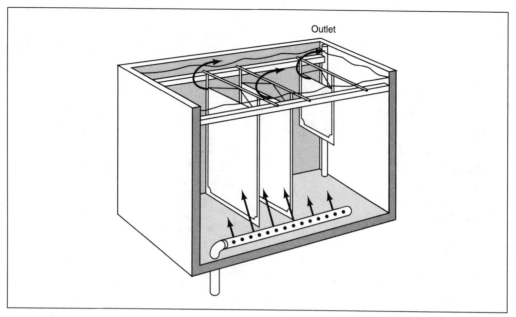

Outlet

Figure 9-16 Single wash compartment

Some processors provide a finished film in as little as ninety seconds. The most important advantage is the constant control over chemical temperature and chemical strength. Chemicals used in automatic processing are more concentrated than in the manual process, and a higher temperature is used.

Automatic processing systems include transport, water, recirculation, replenishment, and dryer systems. Each will be discussed briefly.

Transport System. The transport system, consisting of rollers, transport racks, and drive motors, moves the film through the chemical solutions. It also serves to continuously agitate the chemicals, which prevents settling of the solutions. The transport system begins at the feed tray located in the darkroom. As the film is gently pushed on the feed tray, rollers grip the edge and begin moving it through the processor, Figure 9-19. Microswitches located at the entry to the feed tray detect the film size and start the automatic chemical-replenishment pump. The rate at which the film is transported through the processing tanks is very carefully controlled by the roller system. Roller subassembly consists of one-inch-diameter transport rollers and three-inch master rollers. Most of the rollers, except for those at the feed tray entry, are located within a rack. This allows for easy removal to clean and service the assembly. The transport system is powered by a motor whose time is set to the manufacturer's specifications.

Basic Manual Processing of X-ray Film

Timer and thermometer: These are essential and must be accurate. Check the temperature of the developer and adjust it if necessary. Rinse the thermometer afterwards. Set the timer for the desired period of development based on the temperature of the developer. See the chart below.

Safelighting: Be sure that lamps are in good condition and located at least 4 feet (1.2 meters) from working surfaces. Use a KODAK GBX-2 Safelitht Filter, or equivalent, for all films. Maximum wattage of bulb—7½ watts for KODAK SB Film; 15 watts for all other films listed on this chart.

Chemicals: In preparing solutions, follow directions packaged with the chemicals exactly. Stir gently and thoroughly using separate paddles for each solution to avoid contamination. Be sure to replenish solutions properly.

Handling Film: Do not bend the film. Handle it only by the edges to avoid finger marks or abrasions when attaching it to a hanger. Separate hangers in solutions so that films will not touch one another or the tank wall.

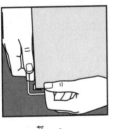

1 LOAD FILM ON HANGER
Turn out lights. Attach film carefully to hanger of proper size. Attach lower corners first. Avoid finger marks, scratching, and bending.

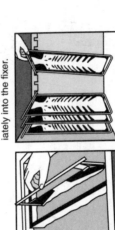

2 IMMERSE FILM IN DEVELOPER
Completely immerse film. Do it smoothly and without pause to prevent streaking. Tap hanger sharply to dislodge air bubbles. Start timer. Do not agitate.

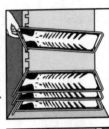

3 DRAIN OUTSIDE DEVELOPER TANK
When alarm rings, lift hanger out quickly. Then drain film for a moment into the space between tanks. For faster drainage, lift hanger.

4 RINSE THOROUGHLY
Rinse film for 30 seconds in fresh, running water or KODAK Indicator Stop Bath at 60-85°F (15-30°C). Agitate continuously. If water is used, lift film and drain well; if an acid stop bath, plunge film immediately into the fixer.

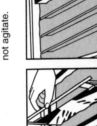

5 FIX IMMEDIATELY
Immerse films. Fix for 2-4 minutes in KODAK GBX Fixer and Replenisher at 60-85°F (15-30°C). Agitate 5 seconds every 30 seconds. Allow excess fixer to drain back into fixer tank.

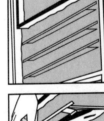

6 WASH COMPLETELY
Place in a tank of clean running water (8 volume changes/hour):
- KODAK Blue Brand Film —20 min.
- KODAK SB, Single-Coated Medical/Green-Sensitive, and PHOTO-FLURE Films—30 min.
- all other films—5 min.

7 FINALE RINSE
If facilities permit, use a final rinse of KODAK PHOTO-FLO Solution to speed drying and prevent watermarks. Immerse film for about 30 seconds and drain for several seconds.

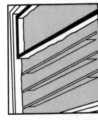

8 PLACE IN DRYER
Place in dryer or rack in a dust-free current of air. Keep films well separated. When dry, remove films from hangers and insert in identified envelopes.

Figure 9-17   Basic manual processing of X-ray film (*Reprinted courtesy of Eastman Kodak Company*)

KODAK Time-Temperature Processing Chart

FOR USE WITH:
Kodak GBX Developer and Replenisher and Kodak GBX Fixer and Replenisher

		KODAK X-ray Films			
		T-MAT	X-OMAT S, X-OMAT RP, X-OMAT L, Single-Coated Medical/Green-Sensitive	GPG, X-OMAT G, Ortho G, Ortho L, BLUE BRAND, X-OMAT Duplicating, Rapid Process Copy, X-OMAT AR	GPB, SB, X-MAT K, MIN-R, PHOTOFLURE	Ortho H
Develop	For time indicated below. **Do not agitate.** Check developer temperature before each use.					
	68°F 20°C	8 Min	7 Min	5 Min	3½ Min	4 Min
	72 22	7	6	4	3	3
	76 24	5	4	3	2	2½
	80 26.5	4	2½	2	1½	2
Rinse	For **30 seconds** in fresh, running water or KODAK Indicator Stop Bath at 60–85°F (15–30°C). **Agitate continuously.**					
Fix	Fix **2–4 minutes** in KODAK GBX Fixer and Replenisher. **Agitate 5 seconds in every 30 seconds.** KODAK *RP* X-OMAT Fixer and Replenisher or KODAK Rapid Fixer may be used.					
Wash	In clean, running water at 60–85°F (15–30°C) with approximately 8 volume changes per hour. Wash for **5 minutes** *except:* BLUE BRAND Film for 20 minutes; SB, Single-Coated Medical/Green-Sensitive, and PHOTOFLURE Films for 30 minutes.					
Dry	At room temperature in a dust-free area or a suitable drying cabinet. Temperature not to exceed 120°F (50°C).					

Replenishment instructions are different for each solution.
Follow the specific recommendations for the developer replenisher and fixer replenisher furnished with chemical concentrates.

Figure 9-18 Kodak time-temperature processing chart *(Reprinted courtesy of Eastman Kodak Company)*

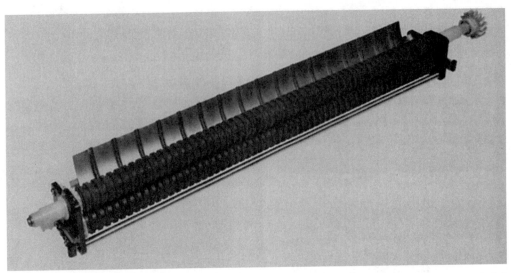

Figure 9-19 Crossover rack with ribbed guide shoes *(Reprinted courtesy of Eastman Kodak Company)*

Water System. The water system washes the film and helps to stabilize the temperature of the solutions. Incoming water into the processor is maintained by a thermostatic regulating device.

Recirculation System. The recirculation pump blends and mixes the developer and fixer solutions with replenishment solution. This is very important for maintaining the proper temperature and chemical-activity level of the solutions. Constant agitation keeps the solutions mixed and in contact with the film.

Replenishment System. Automatic-processing chemicals are replenished by replenishment pumps each time a film enters the feed tray rollers. Manufacturers recommend replenishment rates based on the number of films processed. This method assumes a common density to each film and bases the quantity of replenishment solution upon a known standard of silver halide conversion to metallic silver. Regular checks are required to assure that the replenishment rates are accurate. This process is considered part of a quality control program.

Dryer System. Automatic-processor drying consists of a blower system that disperses heated air around the film as it moves past.

Limited radiographers should be familiar with automatic-processing components. Each manufacturer provides detailed operating and maintenance manuals, and these should be consulted whenever questions arise. Also, most X-ray sales and service companies provide representatives who help answer technical film-processing questions.

Processing films in an automatic processor is a simple task. Exercise 9-9 in the Appendix offers a step-by-step guide to automatic film processing.

Artifacts

Film artifacts are undesirable. They consist of a wide range of extraneous marks and areas of increased or decreased density (darkening) that interfere with the diagnostic value of the radiograph. Table 9-5 provides a list of common artifacts. They are caused by physical, mechanical, and chemical means and may be avoided if proper film handling and storage procedures and appropriate film-processing guidelines are observed. Table 9-6 provides a list of common problems and corrections related to handling and processing X-ray film. After films are processed they should be checked for artifacts. If artifacts are visible, the cause or source should be determined and corrected, Figures 9-20 through 9-23.

TABLE 9-5 ▪ Artifacts and Sources

ARTIFACT	SOURCE
Brown Stain	From old or oxidized developer (too much air has mixed with the solution)
Multicolored Stain	From poor rinsing
Yellowish Film	From exhausted or weakened fixer solution
Milky-white Film	From incomplete washing time
Streaking	From solutions that have not been stirred well or films not agitated well, films not rinsed adequately, poor circulation in automatic processor, and/or withdrawing film after it had started through the entrance assembly of the processor. In manual processing, check the wire hanger clips for chemical residue. Clean with a stiff brush.
Crinkle Marks	From kinking the film during handling
Reticulation	Weblike marks that appear in the emulsion when there are extreme differences in the processing solutions.
Hesitation Marks	From automatic processor when the film hesitates or stops, causing increased density lines across the film.
Guide Shoe Marks	From automatic processor when film guide racks are not lined up properly with the rollers closest to them.

TABLE 9-6 ▪ Handling and Processing X-Ray Film: Common Problems and Corrections

PROBLEM	CAUSE	CORRECTION
Radiograph too dark	1. Overexposure	1. Reduce exposure
	2. Overdevelopment	2. Adjust development time (manual); Check temperatures of water and solutions (automatic)
	3. Concentrated replenishment	3. Adjust replenishment
Radiograph too light	1. Underexposure	1. Increase exposure
	2. Underdevelopment	2. Adjust development time (manual); Check temperatures of water and solutions (automatic)
	3. Exhausted replenishment	3. Adjust replenishment
Fog on radiograph	1. Chemical vapor exposure	1. Store film away from hydrogen sulfite, hydrogen peroxide, terpene, mercury
	2. Storage temperatures too high or humidity too high	2. Store film in appropriate place, temperature
	3. Expiration date on film has passed	3. Regularly rotate film stock and use film before expiration date
	4. Safelight exposure	4. Use recommended filter color, bulb wattage, and location of safelight from film-loading bench
	5. X-ray exposure	5. Store film in appropriate place
	6. Pressure	6. Do not apply pressure or stack stored film boxes

TABLE 9-6 ▪ (Continued)

PROBLEM	CAUSE	CORRECTION
Black circular spots	Developer on film before development	Avoid developer splashes on film
White circular spots	Fixer on film before development	Avoid fixer splashes on film
Branched black marks	Static electricity discharge	Use proper film-handling procedures; Avoid clothing that contains excessive static build-up, such as nylon
Crescent-shaped black marks	Bend in the film after exposure	Use proper film-handling procedures
Crescent-shaped white marks	Bend in the film before exposure	Use proper film-handling procedures
Yellow or brown stains	Exhausted developer; exhausted fixer	Replace solution

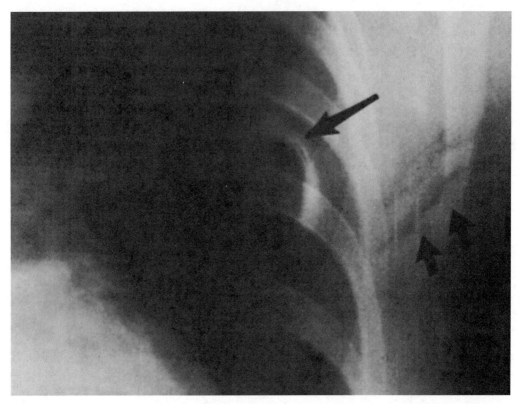

Figure 9-20 Both images on this radiograph were caused by mishandling of the film. The single arrow demonstrates a *crinkle mark*, which can occur if the film is bent. The double arrows show an artifact caused by pressure on the surface of the film.

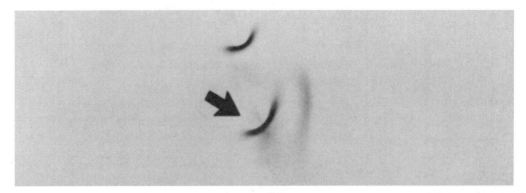

Figure 9-21 Kink, crinkle, or half-moon artifact caused by mishandling of the film. A white crinkle mark is caused by bending the film prior to exposure. A black crinkle mark is caused by bending the film after exposure and prior to processing.

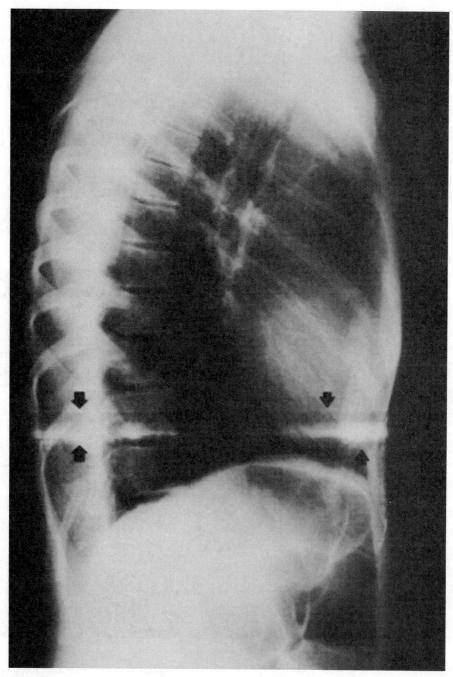

Figure 9-22   Pressure artifact resulting from closing the drawer of the film bin on the sheet of film

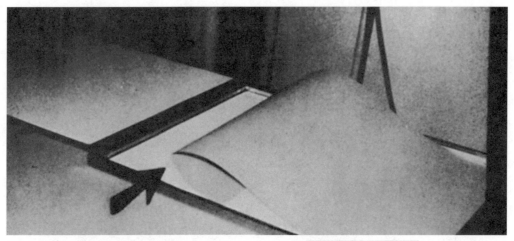

(A)

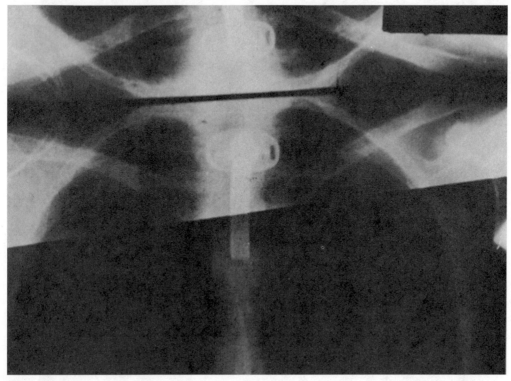

(B)

Figure 9-23   (A) A sheet of film may be accidentally loaded into the cassette in a folded position; (B) The artifact in this radiograph resulted from loading the film into the cassette in a folded position.

AUTOMATIC-PROCESSOR MAINTENANCE

Automatic processors, like any electromechanical equipment, must have regular service and repair. Processor maintenance consists of the usual daily, weekly, and monthly care as well as preventive and nonscheduled maintenance. Generally, limited radiographers are not expected to perform preventive or repair maintenance; such procedures are usually performed by skilled service people. Radiographers are, however, expected to perform the usual daily processor care, maintain a designated preventive maintenance schedule and records, and recognize the need for nonscheduled repair. Suggestions for daily processor care follow:

- Clean crossover rollers (use water and a nonabrasive, lint-free cloth), Figure 9-24.
- Observe all moving parts for wear. Report anything unusual to immediate supervisor.
- Check level of replenishment solutions in storage tanks.
- Drain the wash tank and offset the processor lid at night (this prevents the build up of algae in the tanks).

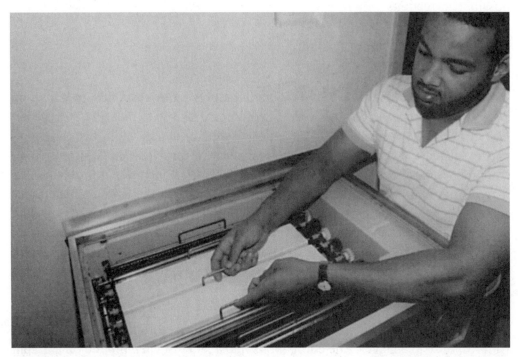

Figure 9-24 This radiographer is removing and cleaning crossover rollers from an automatic processor as part of a daily maintenance routine.

Preventive maintenance should be regularly scheduled. Each manufacturer will suggest a planned program that should be followed. Consult with company representatives or X-ray sales and service personnel to determine the best schedule to follow.

Nonscheduled maintenance is the most dreaded because it means a mechanical or electrical failure within the processor. The number of these incidents can be reduced with a regular preventive maintenance program. How does one know if something is wrong? Generally, automatic-processor problems will first become evident on the films. Unusual scratches, lines, marks, or improper processing of the films will be noticed. Also, some problems will be noticed first as an unusual operating sound. Limited radiographers are not expected to diagnose such problems, but before making a service call, it is important for the radiographer to note any detail noticed, e.g., nature of the problem, visual appearance of films processed, unusual sounds, or signs of leaks or mechanical failure. It is also a good idea to check all temperature and chemical controls before reporting the problem. Table 9-6 lists common film handling and processing problems and possible corrections.

SENSITOMETRY

Sensitometry is the study of how radiographic film responds to radiation exposure and processing conditions. Sensitometry is used to measure and predict how film density will change as radiation exposure factors and processing conditions change. By monitoring these responses, it provides early detection of equipment malfunctions before they can cause serious operational problems that may result in repeat of patient examinations. Changes in the film characteristics can be easily detected by sensitometry when radiation exposure and processing conditions are constant. Changes in processing conditions may also be identified when film-screen system and radiation exposure factors are constant. Sensitometry measurements include those visibility factors of density, contrast, and fog.

A characteristic curve, sometimes called H & D curve and first used in 1890 for photography analysis by Hurter and Duffield, is used to measure and predict film response to changes. The curve looks like a letter S when plotted on a graph, Figure 9-25. The graph is plotted by exposing a film and plotting the density levels against a logarithm of the various exposure levels.

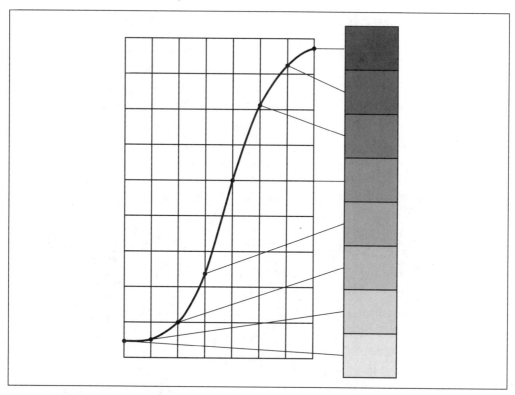

Figure 9-25   The H & D curve *(Reprinted courtesy of Eastman Kodak Company)*

Sensitometry Methods

There are three methods of performing sensitometry: step-wedge pentrometer and medium exposure, sensitometer exposure, and pre-exposed sensitometry strips. Most limited radiographers will be involved with only the third and easiest method of sensitometric measurement; thus, this is the only method that will be described.

In the procedure for pre-exposed sensitometry test strips, the strips are purchased and are stored in the film bin. When processed, the strips will have areas of increasing density. The processed strips are analyzed in a densitometer, an instrument with a light-sensing device. The amount of light transmitted through each segment on the strip is measured. A characteristic curve should result when this information is recorded and analyzed. Strips are regularly processed and the densities evaluated. This is a very common, widely used method today. Sensitometry application to film processing will be discussed in more detail with radiographic exposures.

SILVER RECOVERY

Silver, a treasured metal, can be recovered from fixer processing chemicals. Silver can also be reclaimed from scrap film and purged radiographic films. Why recover silver? Silver recovery is one way to salvage a scarce natural resource and also provides a small monetary return. The unexposed silver halide is dissolved in the fixer as the radiograph progresses through the film-processing cycle. There are two common methods used to recover silver from the fixer solution: metallic replacement and electrolytic recovery, Figure 9-26.

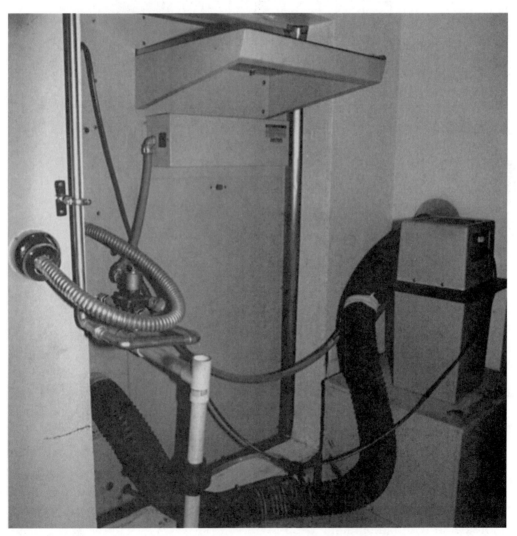

Figure 9-26   Silver-recovery system attached to an automatic processor

Metallic replacement removes silver from the used fixer solution by chemically replacing silver with another metal. As the metal dissolves, the silver moves to the bottom of the container and is removed.

Electrolytic recovery uses electrodes placed in the fixer tank. An electric current causes the silver to attach to one of the electrodes.

To determine which silver recovery system to use, consult with the processor manufacturer or an X-ray service company. Some X-ray service companies will perform routine processor maintenance and cleaning in return for the silver recovery profit.

REVIEW QUESTIONS

1. What are the two main parts of radiographic film?
    a) emulsion and gelatin
    b) gelatin and silver halide crystals
    c) film base and gelatin
    d) film base and emulsion
2. A cassette or direct exposure film holder must be
    a) lighttight
    b) airtight and lightweight
    c) adhesive and airtight
    d) waterproof and fluorescent
3. To reduce excessive radiation exposure to the patient, the following combination should be used:
    a) screen film and cassette
    b) direct exposure film and cassette
    c) direct exposure film and cardboard holder
    d) screen film and cardboard holder
4. The active (phosphor) layer of an intensifying screen
    a) converts X-ray photons to visible light
    b) makes the screen lightproof
    c) decreases buildup of static electricity
    d) converts X-ray energy into light energy
5. Rare-earth intensifying screens have the following advantage compared to calcium-tungstate intensifying screens:
    a) provide more visible detail
    b) require less radiation and shorter exposure time
    c) permit shorter exposure time but require more radiation
    d) less costly

6. Select the spectral matching combination which would reduce the patient's radiation dose.
   a) high-speed film and high-speed screen
   b) high-speed film and low-speed screen
   c) low-speed film and high-speed screen
   d) low-speed film and low-speed screen

7. Radiographic film is *not* sensitive to
   a) chemicals
   b) heat
   c) pressure
   d) odors

8. Unexposed silver halide crystals are removed from the film in the _____ stage of film processing.
   a) development
   b) wash
   c) final rinse
   d) fixation

9. The following is *not* a component of the fixer:
   a) reducing agent
   b) preserver
   c) hardener
   d) acidifier

10. In an automatic processor, the chemicals are agitated by the _____.
    a) replenishment
    b) water
    c) recirculation pump
    d) dryer

11. If a radiograph is fogged, the radiographic density will
    a) increase
    b) decrease
    c) no change
    d) none of the above

12. Radiographic film is more easily fogged
    a) before being loaded into a film holder
    b) after its exposure to X rays but before processing
    c) after processing
    d) after storage
13. The processing solution with an acid ph is
    a) developer
    b) fixer
    c) rinse
    d) wash
14. Fogging of the radiograph produces increased
    a) density
    b) contrast
    c) distortion
    d) recorded detail

REFERENCES

1. *The Fundamentals of Radiography*, 12th ed, p. 34 Health Sciences Markets Division, Eastman Kodak Company, Rochester, New York 14650.
2. Ibid.
3. Sweeney, Richard J., R.T., F.A.S.R.T., *Radiographic Artifacts: Their Cause and Control*. Philadelphia: J. B. Lippincott Company, 1983.

BIBLIOGRAPHY

Carroll, Quinn B. *Fuch's Radiographic Exposure, Processing and Quality Control*. 5th ed. Springfield, Illinois: Charles C. Thomas Publisher, 1993.

Cullinan, Angeline, R. T. (R), F.A.S.R.T. *Producing Quality Radiographs*. Philadelphia: J. B. Lippincott Company, 1987.

Haus, Arthur G. *Film Processing in Medical Imaging*. Madison, Wisconsin: Medical Physics Publishing, 1993.

Pizzutiello, Robert J., and John Cullinan (Eds.). *Introduction to Medical Radiographic Imaging*. Rochester, New York: Eastman Kodak Company, 1993.

Selman, Joseph. *The Fundamentals of X-ray and Radium Physics*. 7th ed. Springfield, Illinois: Charles C Thomas, Publisher, 1985.

Chapter **10**

Evaluation of Radiographic Quality: Image Evaluation

Chapter Outline

Introduction
Image-Quality Considerations
Preparation of Image Production
Radiographic-Film Processing
Identification of Corrective Factors for Poor Radiographic Quality
  Radiographic-Image Evaluation

Objectives

Upon completion of the chapter, the student will meet the following objectives by verifying knowledge of the facts and principles presented through oral and written communication at a level deemed competent.

1. Identify a minimum of four factors that control film quality.
2. List some actions that are generally acceptable when adjustments are required on radiographs that are too dark or too light.
3. Identify appropriate steps for proper radiographic positioning technique that affect film quality.
4. List five basic steps that relate to maintaining proper processing technique.
5. Identify and describe an appropriate method for critique of exposure factors for evaluation of radiographic quality.

   TASKS (see Appendix):
1. Given example radiographs showing both acceptable and poor radiographic quality, evaluate the radiographs according to appropriate criteria.
2. Given radiographs showing processing factors used, identify the problem and list probable causes and corrective actions.

INTRODUCTION

Evaluation of radiographic quality is a process of visually assessing the image recorded on a film. When we look at a black and white photograph, we automatically look for detail in a person's face, a building, a landscape, and so forth. If the photograph is too dark, too light, or motion is seen, information is lost.

The radiographer must possess the appropriate knowledge and skills to visualize, inspect, and determine that technical qualities of the radiographic image are satisfactory. This chapter will address photographic qualities related to visual concepts of a recorded radiographic image. Visual inspection of the finished radiographic image under proper illumination (placed on a viewbox) will reveal most black-and-white (photographic) deficiencies related to too much or too little milliampere seconds (mAs), kilovoltage peak (kVp), or source-to-image distance receptor (SID).

Evaluation of the radiographic image includes multiple factors that are referred to in sum as *photographic effect* or *radiographic quality*. These factors have been dealt with fundamentally in Chapter 8 under exposure factors mA, time, mAs, kVp, and SID. Relative to radiographic quality, these exposure factors may be discussed in terms of the following areas: 1) image-quality considerations, 2) preparation of image production, and 3) radiographic film processing.

IMAGE-QUALITY CONSIDERATIONS

Most people have difficulty seeing what they are not prepared to see. For example, in a stroll through a black-and-white photographic exhibit in a gallery or museum, many viewers react only in terms of whether they like or dislike the subject of a photograph. Others, who have had training in photography or art, additionally react to the shapes, lines, movement, contrast of light and dark, perspective, etc. Details and the quality of the overall effect, rather than the subject, are probably more important to the trained viewer.

In radiography, through educational preparation, the operator must learn about exposure factors and the often delicate balance and interaction between these factors in order to produce film images and then to evaluate the quality of those images. To assess a radiograph, the radiographer's preparation must include knowledge of the following "chain" of factors, their interplay, and their effects on the finished image: the exact mA, time, and kVp; patient's history and present condition; the centimeter measurement of the body part being examined; the processing time and temperature; and any variation in these factors that may have occurred before or during exposure of the image. Knowing these factors and their interactions is crucial when it becomes necessary to repeat a radiograph. The radiographer who produced the initial image should conduct the second attempt to avoid making the same errors or a different error.

PREPARATION OF IMAGE PRODUCTION

When preparing to produce a radiographic image, the operator should employ a systematic approach in order to avoid mistakes. Simple criteria in the form of a checklist should be followed. Because radiographic quality is affected by improper positioning, these criteria should include steps to avoid poor positioning, which often results in repeating radiographs. Such a checklist should include the following procedures:

1. Carefully read the request for radiographic examination to assure that you are very clear on the doctor's instructions regarding what radiographic procedure(s) has been ordered. If there is doubt, confirm the radiographic procedure with the doctor.
2. Identify the patient by *asking* his/her name. Do not suggest: "Are you Mr. Smith?" Rather, simply ask "What is your name, Sir?" If the patient cannot respond, check the arm band or follow the appropriate procedure according to office or departmental policy.
3. The patient must be placed appropriately, according to certain basic principles of radiographic positioning.
   a. Proper radiographic positioning may be effective only when applied with sound knowledge of human structure.
   b. Prior to examination, the patient must be given proper instructions regarding the radiographic procedure.
   c. The patient must be made comfortable to avoid the interactive pull of muscle strain that can result in motion.
   d. The patient's entire body must be positioned so that alignment is achieved with the part of the anatomy being examined, to avoid a rotated or twisted effect that may obscure structural information.
   e. After proper body position has been obtained, it is essential that the part being examined be immobilized. Effective mobilization devices that tend to reduce motion are sandbags, tape, or compression bands.

(Although the next three checklist items, f–h, do not all pertain to positioning, each step is crucial to production of an image as a whole.)

    f. A film size that adequately includes only the anatomical part being examined is necessary. The part in focus is placed in the image receptor's (film cassette's) center and a small unexposed border around the image at the film's edges (½" to 1½") should be visible. The border indicates exposure limitation.

    g. A very important geometric factor is to place the long axis of the anatomical part being examined parallel to, in the center of, and adjacent to the long axis of the image receptor. This avoids magnification of the structure and/or distortion.

    h. The central ray must be directed perpendicular to the long axis of the image and to the center of the image so that it passes through the center point of the structure.

4. Identify the film inside the image receptor with an appropriate marker (usually lead). Place the marker on top of the receptor in the margins of the film outside the structure. (See 3f.)

5. Measure the part being examined and select the exposure factors—*mAs*, *kVp*, and SID (usually standardized, but check to make sure). Measure the part being examined and *set kVp* unless using automatic exposure.

6. Before making exposure, give the patient final instructions and make a final check of the patient's whole body position. Specifically check the part being radiographed to assure that the position has not changed.

7. While constantly observing the patient through a leaded window, observe the mAs-reading on the control console for correct exposure. Do not hold your head outside the protection booth to talk to the patient during exposure.

8. Return the patient to the waiting area after completion of all films. It is not wise to leave an unstable patient unattended in the room.

9. Check the film after processing and if radiographic quality is visible, release patient.

RADIOGRAPHIC-FILM PROCESSING

You have already learned about what is involved in film processing in Chapter 9. Because film processing, like radiographic image production, also involves a chain of events, it is necessary to observe that certain processing elements are constant at all times under any conditions:

1. The time and temperature of the processor must remain at constant levels. Any change in time of processing or degree of temperature will quickly affect the developer solution. If the temperature decreases, the result will be incomplete development (lighter image); if the temperature increases, development of the image will be darker due to chemicals that are too hot.
2. Processor water flow must be constant and maintained at adequate flow pressure.
3. All hoses to the automatic processor and its replenishment tanks must be open, not kinked or clogged, which can cut off chemical flow.
4. The processor must have a schedule for regular maintenance and preventive maintenance.
5. Processor care is generally coordinated with a processor-maintenance person. Day-to-day care of the processor is the responsibility of the radiographer and any others who are involved in equipment care. See Chapter 9, Radiographic-Film Processing, for further information.

IDENTIFICATION OF CORRECTIVE FACTORS FOR POOR RADIOGRAPHIC QUALITY
Radiographic-Image Evaluation

There are three areas in which the sum of the radiographic image, in terms of photographic effect, may be evaluated: 1) photographic factors, 2) geometric factors, and 3) accurate radiographic position.

The finished radiographic image will appear either correct or incorrect in the eye of the beholder. If the image is incorrect, then the operator must visually determine if the image is photographically deficient in contrast (kVp) or density (mAs), or if the processing is of poor quality.

When the completed radiograph has been placed on the illuminator (viewbox), the contrast and density (discussed in Chapter 8) of the image should be such that all areas in the anatomy are visible. A rule of thumb is that if the image is so dark (black) that nothing is visible, the mAs should be cut back to one-fourth of what was originally used (e.g., reduce from 40 mAs to 10 mAs) and then determine whether or not the film is adequate for exposure. When the image is dark but some anatomy can be seen by using a bright light or spotlight, reduce the mAs by only one-half (e.g., from 40 mAs to 20 mAs).

Unless appropriate preparation for image production has taken place, i.e., the radiographer understands and has carefully selected mAs, kVp, and SID (usually standard), only guesses can be made—trial and error—to correct radiographic technique (density and contrast) of poor quality in a recorded image.

Except in the case of patient motion, geometric factors are seldom a problem because most are standardized. Errors involving blurring or distortion (shape, size) are generally related to improper positioning, incorrect body alignment, misjudgment of the patient size and shape (body habitus), or inexperience. When an image is assessed for quality, consideration should be given to the accuracy of all of the factors used to produce the image. Most often, when the image is of poor quality, overexposure or, less frequently, underexposure is the problem and is usually correctable by an adjustment of the exposure time. However, not all problems may be so simply corrected. Tables 10-1 and 10-2 provide some basic category information that may be useful for evaluating the quality of radiographic images.

TABLE 10-1 ▪ Radiographic Quality Chart–Image Visibility

DENSITY: Overall Image Appears Overexposed or Underexposed
Factors to be considered:

mAs: Review the amount of mAs used

kVp: Review measurement of the part for amount of kVp used (too much scatter)

Processing: Check processor temperature and time (rarely a problem)
                 Check for chemical contamination (fog)

(If the problem is not related to above areas, investigate further.)

CONTRAST: Overall Image Appears Flat and Gray or
                      All Appropriate Structures Are Not Penetrated
Factors to be considered:

kVp: Review the amount of kVp used and part measurement. A flat gray or fogged appearance is usually caused by scattered radiation from excessive kVp.

mAs: Review the amount of mAs used. A gray appearance (added density) may be the result of using too much mAs.

Processing: Check processor temperature. A gray appearance (added density) may also result from processing at a temperature too high.
                       Check for chemical contamination (fog).

TABLE 10-2 ▪ Radiographic Quality Chart– Geometric Factors

IMAGE BLURRING: Image Appears Blurred (Unsharp) on the Processed Radiograph

Factors to be considered:

Patient breathed/moved:
Determine if patient breathed or moved during exposure. If the patient breathed, check the reason and use a faster time, if necessary, to eliminate motion. The most effective recourse against motion is a faster time. Immobilization and sand-bag support should also be considered when motion is a problem.

Film-screen contact:
Although poor screen contact is rare today with the excellent construction of cassettes, it still occurs. When it occurs, the screens must be replaced in the cassette. It is unusual for screen contact to be a problem with cassette sizes other than 14" × 17".

DISTORTION: Shape/Size of Image Appears Distorted

Factors to be considered:

SID/OFD:
If the part is or must be placed away from the film surface, the SID should be increased to reduce magnification of size caused by the increase in part-image receptor distance. The part should be no more than 1½"–2" away from the image receptor at 40" SID or 2½"–3" away from the image receptor at 60" SID.

Tube angulation:
Elongation or foreshortening of the part is usually caused by incorrect alignment of the tube or part. Remember, the part to be examined must be parallel to the plane of the image receptor and the tube directed perpendicularly (no angle) through the center point of the anatomy to be viewed. Whenever possible, it is more desirable to rotate the part and keep the anatomy parallel to the image receptor than to angle the tube through the part.

POSITIONING: The Image Appears to Be Incorrectly Positioned

Factors to be considered:

Relationship of anatomy to the image receptor plane and relationship of the CR (central ray) to the anatomy:
Review exactly how the patient was aligned for proper position and how the part to be examined was aligned with the image receptor plane. Poor positioning is a common error and is usually the result of working hurriedly or not checking the position carefully enough. Remember, only one patient can be done at any given time, so there is no need to rush and make mistakes.

Some problems are basic and relatively common in the production of radiographic images. By now you have probably determined that two of the most likely technique errors include overexposure (too much density) and poor positioning. Most overexposure and poor positioning errors generally occur because of the radiographer's lack of attention to details. Table 10-3 identifies a checklist that will acquaint the student with tasks that need to be applied each time a radiographic image is produced.

TABLE 10-3 ▪ Checklist for Evaluating Radiographic Quality

Student's Name ————————————————

Exposure Factors: mAs (mA/T) ———— kVp ————; AEC ————

Processing: Time ———————— Temperature ————————

Radiographic Procedure(s) Requested:

EVALUATION CRITERIA	YES	NO	CORRECTIVE ACTION
Anatomy centered on film			
All necessary anatomical borders are visible			
Right/Left/Date marker visible			
Adequate density (mAs)			
Adequate contrast (kVp)			
Magnification/distortion visible			
Adequate detail/definition visible			
Gonad shielding visible (if req.)			
Collimation (clear border edge)			
Artifacts/visible			
Appropriate image receptor placement			

Table 10-3 is intended to be general in design. Most radiography programs develop their own checklist for evaluating radiographic quality. The checklist in the table may be modified to adapt to any program.

REVIEW QUESTIONS ────────────────────

1. To evaluate radiographic quality means to
   a) visually assess a recorded image
   b) visually inspect a finished radiograph
   c) visualize, inspect, and determine correct image technique
   d) all of the above

2. The limited radiographer's educational preparation must include knowledge of
   a) mA, time, kVp, SID
   b) patient's history and condition assessment
   c) film processing
   d) all of the above

3. In the preparation of image production, which of the following must be done first?
   a) check room availability
   b) check with doctor
   c) carefully read examination request
   d) identify the patient

4. If an overall image appears overexposed or underexposed, generally the first factor to be considered for corrective action is
   a) kVp
   b) mAs
   c) mA
   d) processing

5. If an image has a flat or gray appearance, the problem most likely will be related to
   a) kVp
   b) mAs
   c) processing
   d) time

6. When all anatomy related to a particular image is not visually penetrated, the problem is most likely
   a) kVp too low
   b) kVp too high
   c) mAs too high
   d) mAs too low

7. A blurred image is most likely the result of
   a) motion
   b) kVp too low
   c) mAs too low
   d) no immobilization
8. The most common problem related to image size or shape is
   a) incorrect SID
   b) incorrect kVp
   c) incorrect positioning
   d) incorrect CR
9. If the image appears too long or too short, the _____ is probably not perpendicular to the structure.
   a) image receptor plane
   b) CR
   c) tabletop surface
   d) tube
10. A slight change in the _____ will be seen on the image results almost immediately when film quality is evaluated.
    a) processor water flow
    b) processor time or temperature
    c) processor replenishment rates
    d) processor preventive maintenance

Chapter **11**

Radiation Biology

Chapter Outline

Objectives

Upon completion of the chapter, the student will meet the following objectives by verifying knowledge of the facts and principles presented through oral and written communication at a level deemed competent.

1. Define common radiation terminology.

   a) Identify two sources of naturally occurring background radiation and man-made radiation.

2. Explain the ionization process as it relates to potential biologic damage in humans.

3. Draw an illustration of an atom that has undergone ionization and label the following:
   a) electric charge of the atom before ionization
   b) electric charge of the atom after ionization
   c) ion
   d) ion pair
4. Differentiate between electromagnetic and particulate radiation.
5. Describe the changes that occur on the cellular level as a result of ionization.
6. Draw an illustration to show what occurs in the target or direct-hit theory and the indirect-hit theory.
7. Discuss how the following factors influence biologic damage: 1) type of radiation; 2) amount of radiation received; 3) dose rate; 4) whole body or specific body part exposure.
8. Compare and contrast short-term and long-term radiation-induced biologic effects.
9. Compare and contrast somatic effects and genetic effects of radiation.
10. Recall three factors influencing biologic radiosensitivity.

INTRODUCTION

Radiation biology is a branch of the biological sciences concerned with the effects of ionizing radiation on living organisms. By ionizing radiation we mean the types of electromagnetic and particulate radiation discussed in Chapter 5. These are summarized in Table 11-1.

TABLE 11-1 ▪ Types of Ionizing Radiation

PARTICULATE RADIATION

Source: Originates from the disintegration of the nucleus of radioactive atoms. Particles travel through space as alpha or beta particles.

ELECTROMAGNETIC RADIATION

Source: Gamma rays originate from the disintegration of the nucleus of radioactive atoms. X rays originate from X-ray tube production.

Gamma rays and X rays travel through space at the speed of light, and have no mass or charge.

TYPES OF IONIZING RADIATION

There are many forms and sources of radiation. Some types of radiation, such as light from an ordinary light bulb, usually do not adversely affect humans (these are classified as non-ionizing); others, such as X rays, may be harmful. X rays are a type of ionizing radiation. Ionizing radiation causes changes in some of the atoms it passes through, causing them to separate into electrically charged positive or negative particles called ions. This ability to ionize the atoms of cells can make ionizing radiation harmful to living organisms.

Understanding the process of ionization is the key to understanding the harmful biologic effects of ionizing radiation and to recognizing the radiographer's responsibility in minimizing radiation exposure to patients and themselves.

Humans have always been exposed to environmental or naturally occurring background radiation, Table 11-2. Background radiation comes from the sun,

---

TABLE 11-2 ▪ Average Annual Radiation Exposure of U.S. Population Based on NCRP 93

Overall average annual exposure is 360 mrem and all percentages listed are percentages of 360 mrem.

CATEGORY	SOURCE	PERCENTAGE
295 mrem Natural Background		**82%**
	198 mrem Radon	55%
	97 mrem Cosmic, terrestrial, internal	27%
65 mrem Man-Made		**18%**
	40 mrem Medical X-rays	11%
	14 mrem Nuclear medicine	4%
	11mrem Consumer products	3%
Other		
	1.1 mrem Occupational	.3%
	1.1 mrem Fallout	.3%
	0.4 mrem Nuclear fuel cycle	0.1%
	0.4 mrem Miscellaneous	0.1%

Adapted from data found in National Council on Radiation Protection (NCRP 93).

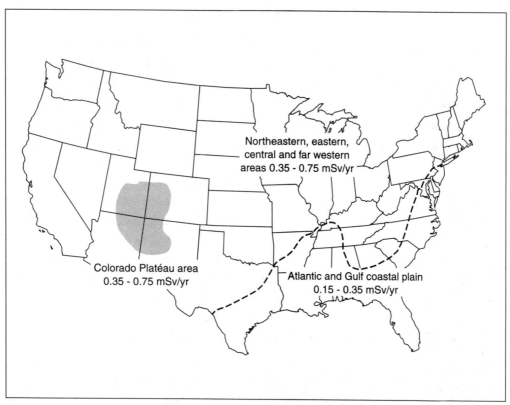

Figure 11-1   Natural background radiation variation in the United States

stars, and from naturally occurring radioactive materials in the soil and water. The actual amount of background radiation varies with the geographic area, its soil and rock composition, and its elevation above sea level, Figure 11-1. Humans receive more radiation exposure at high elevations because there is less atmospheric filtering of the radiation from outer space, called cosmic rays. For example, an individual living in Denver, Colorado, will receive twice the environmental cosmic radiation as an individual living at sea level.

A second major source of environmental radiation comes from naturally occurring radioactive materials, such as uranium, present in the ground, water, and air.

The amount of radiation exposure an individual receives depends on four factors: type of radiation, amount of radiation received, length of time exposed, and the specific parts of the body exposed. These are the underlying bases for radiation-protection measures and will be a basis for risk factors discussed in this chapter and radiation-protection procedures discussed in Chapter 12.

ARTIFICIAL SOURCES OF RADIATION

Since the 1890s, when Roentgen discovered X rays, scientists have been experimenting with ionizing radiation. Much of the knowledge about the harmful effects of radiation has been gathered as a result of the human health consequences from various uses. From the early application of ionizing radiation for diagnostic imaging and treatment of disease to the use of radium for luminous watch dials, the effects and consequences have led to our current focus on exposure reduction and discrimination in applications. Today, radiation sources may be found in nuclear power plants, atomic weapons, ionization-type smoke detectors, airport luggage screening, and in many industrial and commercial applications. The annual average dose of radiation received by humans from medical procedures is much less than the dose received from environmental sources. For example, the average annual radiation exposure of the U.S. population, based on the NCRP 93 Report, is 40 millirems from medical X-rays and 295 millirems from natural background radiation (see Table 11-2).

INTERACTION OF RADIATION WITH MATTER

The effects of radiation on living organisms are a result of the ionizations that occur at the atomic level. During ionization, an electron(s) is removed from its energy shell resulting in a positively charged atom. The free electron can deposit its energy to surrounding tissue. As a result of ionizations, molecules may be altered causing cellular damage that may result in abnormal cell function or loss of cell function. If enough cells have been damaged, the entire organ or organism may display symptoms of radiation damage.

A diagnostic X-ray beam passing through living matter will result in ionization in the cells comprising the matter. Because this interaction and ionization are random, some X rays will pass through matter without interacting. When interaction does occur, X-ray photons will give up their energy to atoms during the interaction, thus altering the atom. The interaction between the X-ray photons and the living matter resulting in energy transfer is called absorption or absorbed dose. The greater the absorbed dose, the greater the possibility of biologic effect. Because there is differential absorption of X rays in body structures of different densities, X rays can be used to visualize these body structures. For example, X rays are absorbed preferentially in bone as compared to soft tissue, thus producing the traditional radiographic image. Attenuation of the X-ray beam refers to any process that prevents X-ray photons from reaching the patient or the radiographic film. Both absorption and scatter, or redirection of an X-ray photon after it has interacted with an object, are factors affecting attenuation.

There are five types of interactions between X rays and matter (Table 11-3):

TABLE 11-3 ▪ Types of Interactions	
TYPE	**CHARACTERISTICS**
Coherent	Also called classical or Thompson's
	Produced by low-energy X-ray photons
	Electrons are not removed but vibrate due to deposit of energy from the photon
	As the electrons vibrate, they emit energy equal to the incoming photon. The energy travels in a path slightly different from the original photon
Photoelectric	Photon absorption interaction
	Incoming X-ray photon strikes a K-shell electron
	Energy of X-ray photon transferred to electron and X-ray photon ceases to exist
	Vacancy hole in K shell is filled by electrons from outer shells, releasing energy which creates low-energy characteristic photons
	This type of interaction results in increased patient radiation dose
Compton	Also called modified scattering
	Incoming X-ray photon strikes a loosely bound, outer-shell electron
	X-ray photon transfers part of its energy to the electron
	Electron is removed from orbit as a scattered electron
	Ejected electrons may ionize other atoms or recombine with an ion needing an electron
	Photon scatters in another direction, with less energy
Pair Production	Ionization does not occur but the photon has scattered Does not occur in diagnostic radiography
	Involves an interaction between the incoming photon and the nucleus of the atom

1. Coherent (Classical or Thompson's) Scattering
2. Photoelectric Effect
3. Compton Effect
4. Photodisintegration
5. Pair Production

Coherent Scattering

Coherent scattering, also called classical or Thompson's scattering, occurs when a low-energy X ray interacts with an atom, Figure 11-2. The target atom becomes energized or "excited" and releases this extra energy as a scattered photon having a wavelength and energy equal to the energy of the original X-ray photon. This released photon is different from the direction of the original X-ray photon; thus it is scattered. In this form of scattering, no energy transfer occurs, and therefore no ionization occurs. Coherent scattering generally occurs in low kVp ranges; however, some occurs throughout the diagnostic kVp range, and is responsible for some small amount of radiographic-film fog.

Photoelectric Effect

The photoelectric effect or interaction occurs when the incident X-ray photon gives up all of its energy to an inner-shell electron, Figure 11-3. When this occurs, an electron, called the photoelectron, is ejected from the atom, usually

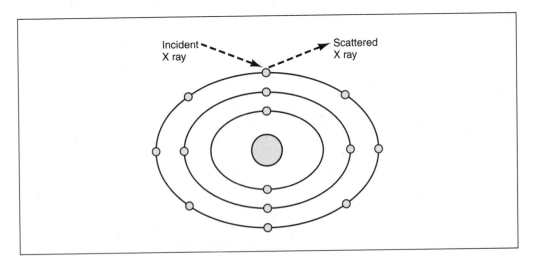

Figure 11-2 Coherent scattering

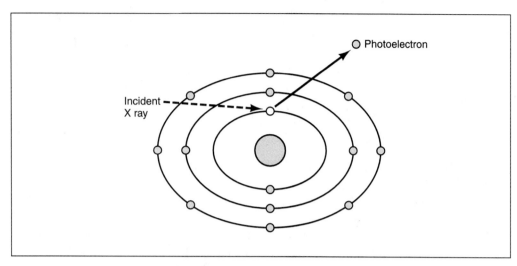

Figure 11-3 Photoelectric effect

from the inner K or L shell, leaving a vacancy or "hole" to be filled in the shell. When an inner-shell electron is removed from an atom, the resulting vacancy is filled by an electron from an outer shell. When an outer-shell electron fills an inner-shell vacancy, an X-ray photon may be emitted from the atom. This type of X ray is called characteristic radiation. Therefore, two types of secondary radiation result from a photoelectric interaction: characteristic X rays and photo-electrons.

Compton Effect

Compton scattering, first described in 1922 by physicist A. H. Compton, is the most common type of X-ray interaction in diagnostic radiology and is responsible for most scattered radiation. Compton scattering occurs when an X-ray photon interacts with an electron in the outer orbital shell of an atom. The outer-shell electron, called a Compton electron, is ejected from the atom and results in ionization of the atom, Figure 11-4. As a result of the interaction, the X-ray photon is redirected, with decreased energy and a longer wavelength. The scattered X-ray photon and the Compton electron have the energy to cause additional ionizing interactions with other atoms. Because Compton-scattered X-ray photons may be deflected in any direction, they are of special concern in radiation protection. Those scattering back in the direction of the incident X ray are referred to as backscatter radiation.

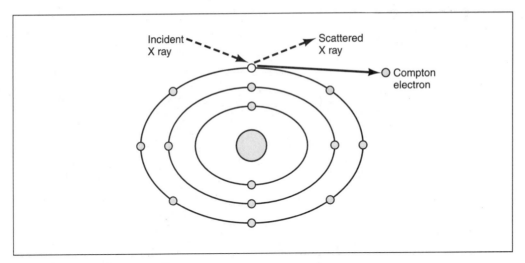

Figure 11-4   Compton effect

Compton scatter radiation, like most scattered radiation, does not contribute to the diagnostic image. Rather, it causes radiographic-film fog and requires the use of lead shielding for protection of the radiation operator and patient.

Photodisintegration

This interaction occurs when a high-energy X-ray photon strikes the atomic nucleus, causing a nuclear fragment to be ejected. This process only occurs with very high energy X-rays and is unlikely to occur in diagnostic radiography.

Pair Production

Pair production is unlikely to occur in the energy ranges used in diagnostic radiology. In this interaction, the incoming photon has sufficient energy to interact with the nucleus of an atom of the irradiated object. This interaction causes the incoming photon to disappear, and in its place two electrons appear, one positively charged and called a positron, and one negatively charged.

CELL ANATOMY

The cell is the basic component of all living organisms. Each cell is a single functioning unit, capable of performing the processes essential for life. A single cell reacts to stimuli, ingests and metabolizes nutrients, synthesizes new materials, excretes wastes, and reproduces. Cells are involved in an ongoing process of obtaining and converting energy; and whatever threatens a cell's existence, in essence, poses a threat to the entire organism.

Collections of cells form tissue and tissues form organs. Organs with similar functions are called systems, Figure 11-5.

The cell has three basic parts: membrane, cytoplasm, and nucleus. The cell membrane is permeable, that is, it allows substances to pass into and out of the cell. The cytoplasm is a watery substance inside the cell. It contains many structures referred to as organelles, whose functions include receiving and converting raw materials into energy. The nucleus, separated from the cytoplasm by a double-walled membrane, consists of fluid (the nucleoplasm) in which the nucleolus and the chromatin material are found. The nucleolus is composed of ribonucleic acid (RNA), and deoxyribonucleic acid (DNA) in the chromatin. The RNA and DNA direct the activities that maintain cell life. Chromosomes that transmit the genetic code of hereditary information are composed of DNA. DNA is a complex molecule that is the carrier of the genetic code of the organism.

Cell division or multiplication is controlled by the nucleus. Two types of cell division occur: mitosis and meiosis. Genetic cells, such as spermatogonium, undergo meiosis; all other cells in the human body undergo mitosis.

In mitosis, the cell divides to form two cells. Mitosis occurs in five phases: interphase, prophase, metaphase, anaphase, and telophase.

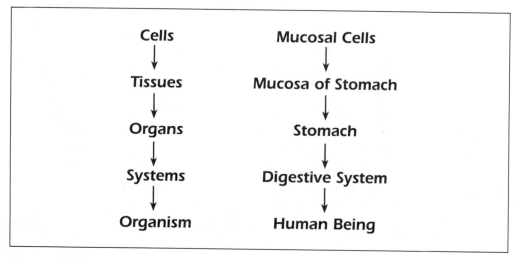

Figure 11-5   The organizational structure of a biological organism

Meiosis, or reduction division, differs from mitosis in that during cell division, the two identical cells produced each contain only one-half of the usual forty-six chromosomes.

Four things may happen when radiation strikes a cell: 1) it may pass through without damage to the cell; 2) it may damage the cell but the cell partially repairs the damage; 3) it may damage the cell so that the cell fails to repair itself but reproduces in damaged form; and 4) it may kill the cell.

RADIOSENSITIVITY

The Law of Bergonié and Tribondeau attempts to explain the basis of living-tissue radiosensitivity. The law states the following:

1. Immature, nonspecialized cells are most radiosensitive. Mature, specialized cells are most radioresistant.
2. Cells with a high metabolic level are radiosensitive.
3. Cells that are rapidly growing and dividing are radiosensitive.
4. Immature tissues and organs are radiosensitive.

Several physical factors should be considered in the determination of radio-sensitivity: 1) linear energy transfer, 2) relative biologic effectiveness, 3) dose fractionation and protraction, and 4) individual biologic factors.

Absorbed Dose

The human body consists of many different types of matter each having their own atomic structure. If it were not for these differences, production of a diagnostic radiograph would not be possible. The anatomic structural differences seen on a radiograph result from X-ray interaction with various tissue within the anatomic part. As X rays pass through bodily tissue, they may interact with the atoms or they may exit without interacting. During this travel through the tissue, some or all of the X-ray energy may be transferred to the tissue. This transfer of energy is called absorption. The amount of X-ray energy absorbed per unit mass is called absorbed dose. Biologic damage is directly related to absorbed dose.

> **The amount of energy absorbed by human tissue depends on the following:**
>
> (1) Atomic number of the tissue or object being X-rayed
>
> (2) Energy of the X ray. For example, bone tissue has a higher atomic number (13.8) than does soft tissue (7.4).

In diagnostic kilovoltage ranges of 30 to 150 kVp, bone tissue will absorb more X-ray energy than soft tissue or fat tissue.

- *As the atomic number of the irradiated tissue increases, the absorbed dose increases.*
- *As the X-ray energy decreases, and the resultant wavelength increases (becomes longer), the absorbed dose to the tissue increases.*

Absorbed Dose Equivalent

Absorbed dose equivalent is an expressive method to calculate the effective absorbed dose for all types of ionizing radiation. It is known that not all types of radiation are equal in their ability to cause biologic damage to living tissue. For example, 25-radiation absorbed dose (rad) of fast neutrons would result in more biologic damage than 25-radiation absorbed dose (rad) of X ray. The method of calculating absorbed dose equivalent considers this difference in potential to cause biologic damage in using the modifying or quality factor (QF). The following formula is used to calculated the absorbed dose equivalent.

ADE (absorbed dose equivalent) = AD (absorbed dose) × QF (quality factor)

Gamma rays, beta particles (high speed electrons), and X rays have a quality factor value of 1 since they produce nearly the same biological effects in body tissue for equal absorbed doses.

Linear energy transfer or LET is the unit of measurement of the amount of the average energy deposited in tissue per unit of track or path length. This concept is important in determining potential biologic tissue damage from ionizing radiation.

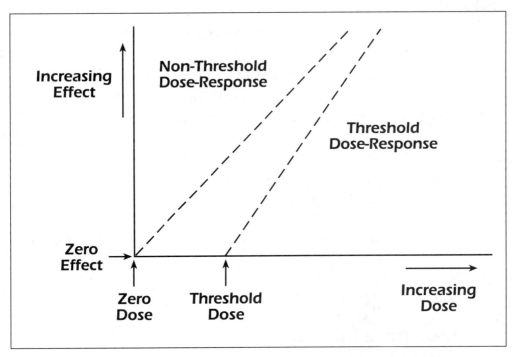

Figure 11-6 A theoretical depiction of the radiation dose-response relationship

Dose-Response Relationship

A dose-response relationship refers to a point or level of exposure (dose) at which a response or reaction first occurs, Figure 11-6. The relationship between radiation and some biologic responses is a linear, non-threshold relationship. This means that any amount of ionizing radiation, no matter how small, may cause a biologic effect (response). The linear, non-threshold relationship model indicates that there is no amount of radiation exposure that is safe. It is assumed that all ionizing-radiation exposure presents the potential to cause biologic effect. Therefore, any such exposure requires the consistent use and application of radiation-protection measures to protect the patient and those performing the examination.

Linear Energy Transfer (LET)

Linear energy transfer (LET) is a unit of measurement that relates to the quantity of absorbed dose and is an important concept in radiation biology. The amount of ionization that occurs in tissue is directly related to how much energy (absorbed dose) it receives. The biologic damage to tissue coincides with the amount of ionization that occurs. The degree of ionization resulting from various types of electromagnetic radiation is not equal. For example, particulate radiation, such as alpha particles, lose energy quickly as they interact with tissue. This quick loss of energy causes many ionizations in the tissue. Alpha and some of the other particulate radiation are said to be high-LET radiation since they have the potential to cause many ionizations as they interact with tissue.

X rays and gamma rays actually produce more interactions in the tissue; however, when compared to some particulate radiation, such as alpha particles, produce fewer ionizations in tissue and are considered to be low-LET radiation.

The extent of biologic effects is dependent upon:
- **Absorbed Dose (AD)**
- **Absorbed Dose Equivalent (ADE)**
- **Linear Energy Transfer (LET)**
- **Relative Biologic Effectiveness (RBE)**

Relative Biological Effectiveness (RBE)

Biologic damage resulting from radiation interaction with tissue increases as the LET of radiation increases. Many scientists have attempted to quantify different types of radiation as to their biological effectiveness in relation to absorbed dose quantities. This however has proven difficult; therefore, the RBE is not practical for delineating radiation protection dose levels. The quality factor (QF), as previously discussed, is basically a measure of RBE and is used in calculation of the absorbed dose equivalents.

Dose Fractionation and Protraction

If the quantity of radiation (dose) is delivered over a long period of time, the biological effect of the same dose will be less than if it were delivered quickly (short period of time). As the time of delivery of a quantity of radiation is increased, a higher dose will be required to produce the same biological effect. Lengthening of time of the delivery of radiation may be accomplished in two ways, fractionated or protracted.

A protracted dose is one that is delivered continuously but at a lower dose rate. A fractionated dose is one that is delivered at the same dose rate but divided into equal fractional quantities of radiation. Dose fractionation is used in radiation therapy since it allows time for tissue repair and recovery between the doses.

Biologic Factors of Radiosensitivity

Several biological variables must also be considered when discussing cell radiosensitivity. These variables are based on the biological variations of individual organisms.

Age.   Radiosensitivity is highest before birth and until maturity. In diagnostic radiography, according to the Law of Bergonié and Tribondeau, the stage of human growth and development that is most radiosensitive is the embryonic and fetal period. During this human developmental stage, there are a great number of immature, nonspecialized cells which are more susceptible to radiation damage when compared to the adult stage of the human life cycle. This does not mean that the mature adult is resistant to potential biologic damage from radiation exposure; rather the Law of Bergonié and Tribondeau provides a ranking or hierarchy of cell radiosensitivity. This hierarchy is given for the growth stages of human development and ranks cells in order from the least radiosensitive to the most radioresistant. Use of radiation-protection measures are very important for protection of the developing embryo and fetus, all children, and women who may have a likelihood of reproducing.

Sex.   Scientific research indicates that females are approximately 5–10% more radiation-resistant than males.

Oxygen Effect.   Oxygen enhances the effect of ionizing radiation on living organisms by increasing cell sensitivity.

Individual Variation in Response.   Human cells are capable of recovering from radiation damage. The repair mechanism is dependent upon many biological and environmental factors.

There are two means of damaging a cell by radiation. These are the direct effect and the indirect effect. The direct effect refers to radiation interaction in which a photon directly interacts with a "target" or critical DNA molecule. In the indirect effect, a photon strikes a noncritical molecule, usually water, but the noncritical molecule transfers the ionization energy to the critical DNA molecule—an indirect effect. Because the human body is composed of approximately 80% water, it is believed that the greatest percentage of ionizations will occur as interactions between photons and water molecules. When a water molecule is ionized, it separates into free radicals. Free radicals are very chemically reactive forms of ions. A free radical can react quickly with other molecules because it has an electron in the outer-energy shell that does not have a partner (another electron to balance the charge). Since free radicals have an unpaired electron, they are very reactive and can impart some of their excess energy to other molecules. It is this transfer of energy by free radicals that causes biological damage. Free radicals are capable of traveling through the cell and causing biological damage at distances away from their origin.

Radiolysis occurs when a water molecule is ionized, resulting in free ions capable of recombining with other free radicals to form new molecules. The free radicals resulting from the radiolysis, or the breakdown of the molecule have the potential to recombine to form a new water molecule or to combine with other radicals to form new molecules. It is believed that most of the effects of radiation on living organisms are a result of radiolysis or the indirect action caused when a photon interacts with a noncritical molecule, Figure 11-7.

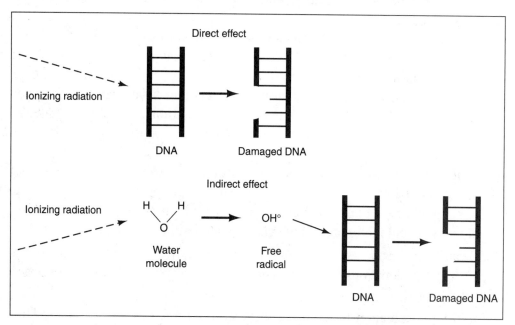

Figure 11-7 The direct and indirect effects of ionizing radiation on DNA

The concept of a sensitive target or key molecule is called the target theory. The target theory states that there is a certain critical target molecule in a cell that must be inactivated in order to damage or kill the cell. Scientists believe that the DNA of a cell represents this target and is the area of the cell vital to cell life and replication.

Biologic effects may be classified as either short-term effects or long-term effects. Biologic effects from radiation fit into one or the other classification, depending upon the length of time it takes for the effect to become evident or demonstrable. As previously discussed, several factors—such as type of radiation, amount of absorbed dose, and body area receiving the exposure—determine the type and intensity of the effect.

Short-term or early effects of exposure to radiation have classically been determined from studies of uranium miners, radium dial painters, survivors of the atomic bombs detonated in Japan during World War II, and survivors of nuclear power plant and nuclear industry accidents.

Short-term effects are found in the acute radiation syndrome, which includes but is not limited to gonadal dysfunctions, epilation (hair loss), depression of the white blood cells, and even death. Clinical signs and symptoms of short-term effects include nausea, vomiting, diarrhea, anemia, leukopenia, hemorrhage, fever, infection, and shock.

Long-term or late effects of radiation may result from small doses of radiation received over a number of years. Long-term effects may also be demonstrated in individuals who have been exposed to a single dose of radiation and have been in a latent period. Examples of long-term effects that have been demonstrated through epidemiologic studies of survivors of radiation exposures include the following:

- *Local tissue effects*. An example of this effect is when the skin undergoes changes in its texture, elasticity, and appearance. It appears dry, chapped, and prematurely aged. Exposed skin may also exhibit an increase in skin lesions, both benign and malignant. These changes are both dose- and time-related.

- *Chromosomal changes*. Chromosome damage may be exhibited as abnormal pairings, translocation, and other phenomena that can result in cell damage and dysfunction.

- *Cataracts*. Radiation-induced cataracts were reported as early as the 1940s. The radiosensitivity of the lens of the eye has been demonstrated to be age-dependent. This means that the older the individual, the more susceptible one is to radiation-induced cataracts.

■ *Life span shortening*. It is suggested that as a result of chromosomal mutations the fitness and life span of an individual acutely exposed will be compromised and/or shortened. For this reason, the amount of radiation delivered in radiographic procedures should always be as low as reasonably possible to obtain the necessary diagnostic information, and radiation-protection measures should always be used.

Somatic and Genetic Effects.   The effects of radiation on living organisms are further classified as somatic or genetic. Somatic effects occur to the individual who has been exposed to ionizing radiation, whereas the genetic effects may not be apparent in the exposed individual but passed on to future generations through genetically damaged chromosomes.

Somatic Effects.   Somatic effects occurring to the living organism may be classified as either early or late somatic effects, depending upon the length of time from the moment of radiation exposure to the first appearance of symptoms.

Early or acute effects are those that appear within minutes, hours, days, or weeks after the initial radiation exposure. Examples of early or acute effects are loss of bone marrow function (hematopoietic syndrome), gastrointestinal syndrome, and central nervous system syndrome.

Late somatic effects are those that appear after a period of months or years after the initial exposure. Late somatic effects may result from an initial high dose of radiation that caused early acute symptoms, and ultimately repair and recovery, or chronic low level doses of radiation received over a long time period. Carcinogenesis is the most important late somatic effect and is difficult to verify statistically because it cannot be distinguished from cancers normally expected in populations.

Radiation Units of Measurement

One of the first units of measurement used for radiation was called the roentgen, after Professor Wilhelm Conrad Roentgen. A roentgen is the unit of measurement of the ionization of air by X rays or gamma rays. The ionizing potential of X rays is now measured in SI units as one coulomb/ kilogram of air.

The units gray (Gy) and sievert (Sv) are used in measuring the effects of radiation on living organisms or materials. The gray expresses the energy per kilogram absorbed as a result of exposure to any type of radiation. One gray is that quantity of radiation that imparts one joule of energy to one kilogram. The gray replaces the rad (*r*adiation *a*bsorbed *d*ose), which expressed the absorption of one erg of energy by one gram of tissue.

The sievert is the unit used to express the quantity of radiation received in an occupational exposure. The gray expresses the quantity of absorbed dose and is an important indicator when considering biologic effects resulting from radiation exposure. But the sievert takes into account the type or source of the radiation and its potential for biologic damage. The sievert has replaced the rem (*r*ad- or *r*oentgen-equivalent *m*an).

The becquerel (Bq) is the unit used to measure radioactivity. A becquerel is a measure of the number of atoms disintegrating (decaying) per second in radioactive material. One becquerel is one radioactive disintegration per second. The becquerel replaces the old unit known as the curie. Table 11-4 shows traditional and international radiation units of measure.

TABLE 11-4 ▪ Radiation Units of Measurement

TRADITIONAL UNIT OF MEASUREMENT	INTERNATIONAL UNIT OF MEASUREMENT	DEFINITION
Roentgen (R)	Coulomb per kilogram (C/kg)	Quantity of charge released as X rays or gamma rays pass through a specific quantity of dry air
RAD (r)	Gray (Gy) *defined as the energy transfer of one joule (J) per kilogram of irradiated object/matter*	Radiation absorbed dose. Indicates the quantity of energy transferred to matter or an object by any type of ionizing radiation
REM (rad-equivalent man) *defined as the unit of the quantity, absorbed dose equivalent of any type of ionizing radiation that produces the same biological effect as one rad of radiation.*	Sievert (Sv) *One sievert equals on hundred rem.*	An absorbed dose in rad may be converted to a rem by use of the quality factor for the type of radiation. Sievert and rem are easily compared by taking the number of rem and dividing by 100 to find the sievert unit

SUMMARY OF HUMAN EXPOSURE TO IONIZING RADIATION

1. Biologic effects are dose-dependent (the greater the amount, the greater the effect).
2. Effects of a given exposure vary from person to person. Predicting exactly how an individual will respond is nearly impossible except at lethal-dose levels.
3. A great amount of radiation delivered over seconds, minutes, or hours is called an acute radiation exposure. Acute doses to the whole body are more dangerous than acute exposure to a specific body part.
4. There is controversy about the long-term effects of low doses of radiation; however, chronic low doses of radiation have been associated with a higher incidence of cancer.

REVIEW QUESTIONS ━━━━━━━━━━━━━━━━

1. Organs with similar functions are called
   a) cells
   b) tissues
   c) organisms
   d) systems
2. Sources of radiation are
   1) man-made
   2) terrestrial
   3) cosmic
      a) 1 and 2
      b) 1 and 3
      c) 2 and 3
      d) 1, 2, and 3
3. In the photoelectric effect, the incident X ray interacts with a(n)
   a) inner-shell electron
   b) proton
   c) nuclear force field
   d) outer-shell electron

4. In the photoelectric effect, the incident X ray
   a) is completely absorbed
   b) is scattered at a lower energy
   c) is scattered at a longer wavelength
   d) is scattered at a higher frequency

5. A cell's sensitivity to radiation is determined by
   1) its degree of specialization
   2) how fast it grows
   3) its state of maturity
      a) 1 and 2
      b) 1 and 3
      c) 2 and 3
      d) 1, 2, and 3

6. Some long-term effects of radiation exposure are
   1) cataracts
   2) life span shortening
   3) epilation
      a) 1 and 2
      b) 1 and 3
      c) 2 and 3
      d) 1, 2, and 3

7. The radiation unit expressed as 1 J/kg is the
   a) roentgen
   b) rad
   c) gray
   d) rem

8. The units of dose that are equivalent are the
   a) rem and rad
   b) roentgen and rem
   c) gray and rem
   d) rem and sievert

9. A unit of radiation exposure is the
   a) rad
   b) roentgen
   c) gray
   d) rem

10. The units of radiation absorbed dose are the
    a) rad and roentgen
    b) roentgen and gray
    c) roentgen and sievert
    d) rad and gray

11. The Law of Bergonié and Tribondeau refers to
    a) living-tissue sensitivity to radiation
    b) the way radiation intensity varies with the distance
    c) the fact that 100 mA at $1/10$ second equals 10 mAs, and 300 mA at $1/30$th of a second equals 10 mAs
    d) none of the above

12. This is the most common type of X-ray interaction in diagnostic radiology
    a) classical scattering
    b) photoelectric
    c) Compton
    d) pair production

13. The term below that is most related to the terms radon, cosmic, and terrestrial radiation is
    a) occupational
    b) medical
    c) consumer
    d) natural

14. Cell sensitivity is determined by
    1. degree of cell specialization
    2. how rapidly the cell grows and divides
    3. the state of maturity of the cell
       a) 1 and 2
       b) 1 and 3
       c) 2 and 3
       d) 1, 2, and 3

15. All of the following refer to dose-response relationship, **EXCEPT**
    a) a level of exposure at which a response first occurs
    b) a relationship between radiation and some biologic response
    c) the same as the law of reciprocity
    d) all of the above

16. The unit of measure of the amount of energy transferred from radiation to tissue as a function of the distance the radiation travels in the tissue is called
    a) reciprocity
    b) attenuation
    c) linear energy transfer
    d) absorption
17. Short-term effects of radiation are likely to result from the following
    a) small doses of radiation received over a number of years
    b) a large dose of radiation received within a short time frame
    c) small incremental doses of radiation
    d) large incremental doses of radiation spread out over many months

BIBLIOGRAPHY

Bushong, Stewart C. *Radiologic Science for Technologists: Physics, Biology, and Protection*, 6th edition, St. Louis, MO: Mosley-Year Book, 1997.

Slatkiewicz-Sherer, Mary Alice, Paul J. Visconti, and E. Russell Retenour. *Radiation Protection in Medical Radiography*, 2nd edition, St. Louis, MO: Mosley-Year Book, Inc. 1993.

Chapter 12

Radiation Protection

Chapter Outline

Objectives

Upon completion of the chapter, the student will meet the following objectives by verifying knowledge of the facts and principles presented through oral and written communication at a level deemed competent.

1. Identify the person who is responsible for evaluating each patient by considering the benefit-versus-risk principle prior to requesting a radiographic examination.
2. Define the term "effective dose equivalent" and state the annual occupational and nonoccupational effective-absorbed-dose-equivalent limit.
3. Explain the ALARA concept and give a minimum of two radiation-protection procedures supportive of the ALARA concept.
4. Summarize the main intent of the 1981 Consumer-Patient Radiation and Safety Act.

INTRODUCTION

The use of X-ray examinations to aid in the diagnosis of disease and injury is often considered to be a standard part of the diagnostic evaluation process. Yet few people realize that the physician must consider several factors before requesting a radiographic examination.

Each time a radiographic examination is indicated, the licensed medical practitioner must consider the potential diagnostic benefits to be gained from the radiographic examination versus the potential biologic harm to the patient resulting from radiation exposure. This decision is often called the benefit-versus-risk principle and must be considered each time a radiologic examination is requested. Once the decision to perform a radiographic procedure has been made by the doctor, it is the radiographer's responsibility to perform the examination and to follow all recognized radiation-protection guidelines. These guidelines consist of cardinal principles and procedures intended to reduce unnecessary radiation exposure to the patient and radiation operator. The main goal of all radiation-protection activities is to keep all radiation exposure *as low as reasonably achievable* (ALARA). This chapter introduces current radiation-protection philosophy, the ALARA *concept, effective-absorbed-dose-equivalent limit guidelines*, and *radiation-protection procedures for the patient and radiation operator*.

EFFECTIVE-ABSORBED-DOSE-EQUIVALENT

Guidelines limiting the amount of radiation received by the general public and those individuals who use radiation in their work (occupational dose) have been established by several international and governmental agencies, Table 12-1.

The agencies named in Table 12-1 determine effective-dose levels and make recommendations that the Nuclear Regulatory Commission (NRC), a national agency, has the responsibility to enforce. There are five regional NRC offices that serve various geographic areas of the United States. Regional NRC offices accept collect telephone calls from employees who wish to register concerns or complaints about conditions or matters within radiologic facilities.

Traditionally, radiation-exposure limits have been expressed as the maximum permissible dose (MPD) of radiation to which the radiation-occupation worker or the general public can be exposed. Over the years, as knowledge of the injurious effects of radiation has increased, the MPD has been decreased, Table 12-2.

However, the MPD is no longer used as the criterion of radiation exposure in

---

TABLE 12-1 ▪ Groups Responsible for Establishing Effective-Absorbed-Dose-Equivalent Limits

(ICRP)	International Commission on Radiological Protection
(NAS-BEIR)	National Academy of Sciences Advisory Committee on the Biological Effects of Ionizing Radiation
(NCRP)	National Council on Radiation Protection and Measurement
(UNSCEAR)	United Nations Scientific Committee on the Effects of Atomic Radiation

---

TABLE 12-2 ▪ Historical Overview of Radiation Exposure Dose Trends

YEAR	APPROXIMATE DAILY DOSE	
1902	100 mSv	10 rem
1925	2.0 mSv	0.2 rem
1928	1.5 mSv	0.15 rem
1936	1.0 mSv	0.1 rem recommended by the United States Advisory Committee on X-Ray and Radium Protection
1959	0.2 mSv	0.02 rem recommended by the National Council on Radiation Protection and Measurements

---

radiation protection. In 1987, the NCRP issued new guidelines for limits on exposure to ionizing radiation based on the dose equivalent. The effective-absorbed-dose-equivalent limits are the product of absorbed radiation dose and the quality factor of the radiation. The quality factor for X rays, gamma rays, beta particles, and electrons is one. The name for the unit of effective-absorbed-dose-equivalent limits is the sievert (Sv). The *dose equivalent* is further defined as the effective dose equivalent for partial-body irradiation of specific organs or tissues and the whole-body. Chapter 11 contains a detailed description of the units used to measure ionizing radiation. For purposes of comparison, a single chest X ray exposes the *patient* to approximately 0.1 mSv (10 mrem).

The recommendations on effective-absorbed-dose-equivalent limits for individuals are based on the general ALARA concept and the negligible individual risk level (NIRL). The NIRL is not a radiation-exposure limit but is the level of risk below which it is unnecessary to control exposure to radiation. However, it may be stated that the NIRL corresponds to an annual effective-absorbed-dose-equivalent limit of 0.01 mSv (0.001 rem).

Effective-absorbed-dose-equivalent limits differ for radiation workers and the general population. They are further modified by reference to specific organ or tissue exposures and embryo-fetus exposures. For occupational exposures, the annual effective-absorbed-dose-equivalent limit is 50 mSv (5 rem). The dose-equivalent limit for the lens of the eye, an especially radiosensitive tissue, is 150 mSv (15 rem). For all other tissues and organs, including bone marrow, breast, lung, gonads, skin, and extremities, the limit is 500 mSv (50 rem). These and other recommendations are summarized in Table 12-3.

TABLE 12-3 ▪ Effective-Absorbed-Dose-Equivalent Limits Summary of NCRP Report #91

OCCUPATIONAL PERSONNEL	ANNUAL DOSE EQUIVALENT	
Effective-absorbed-dose-equivalent limit	50 mSv	(5 rem)
Lens of eye	150 mSv	(15 rem)
All other organs, organ systems, tissue	500 mSv	(50 rem)
Cumulative exposure	10 mSv × age	(1 rem × age)
NONOCCUPATIONAL (General Public)	**ANNUAL DOSE EQUIVALENT**	
Continuous or frequent exposure	1 mSv	(0.1 rem)
Infrequent exposure	5 mSv	(0.5 rem)
Lens of eye, skin, and extremities	50 mSv	(5 rem)
EDUCATION AND TRAINING EXPOSURES	**ANNUAL DOSE EQUIVALENT**	
Effective-absorbed-dose-equivalent limit	1 mSv	(0.1 rem)
Lens of eye, skin, and extremities	50 mSv	(5 rem)
EMBRYO-FETUS EXPOSURES		
Total dose-equivalent limit to term	5 mSv	(0.5 rem)
Dose-equivalent limit in a month	0.5 mSv	(0.05 rem)

The age of the radiation worker is also a factor in exposure limitations. Previously, no one under eighteen years of age was allowed to work with ionizing radiation. The NCRP has stated that for educational and training purposes, radiation workers less than eighteen years old be limited to an annual effective absorbed dose equivalent of 1 mSv (0.1 rem). In addition to annual dose limitations, a cumulative or lifetime dose limitation must be observed. This limit is determined by the age of the radiation worker. The total allowable cumulative exposure is the age (in years) of the worker times 10 mSv (1 rem). For example, a thirty-year-old radiographer is allowed a cumulative exposure of 30 $\times$ 10 mSv or 300 mSv (30 rem).

Guidelines for exposure limitations for the general public are less than those for radiation workers. The effective absorbed dose equivalent for continuous or frequent exposures is 1 mSv (0.1 rem) and for infrequent exposure 5 mSv (0.5 rem).

Embryo-fetal exposures are also considered separately. The total dose-equivalent limit for the embryo-fetus is 5 mSv (0.5 rem) and the dose-equivalent level in a month is 0.5 mSv (0.05 rem).

RADIATION-PROTECTION PROCEDURES

The Patient

The main goal of any radiation-protection procedure is to reduce unnecessary radiation according to the ALARA concept. Reducing unnecessary or excessive radiation exposure is a responsibility shared by everyone involved with radiologic examinations, including the doctor, radiation operator, and all support staff. There are four major areas that relate to reducing radiation exposure: patient preparation, primary-beam limitation, gonadal shielding, and technical factors.

Patient Communication.   The first time when radiation-protection guidelines may be applied is when the examination is requested by the attending physician. It is the attending doctor's responsibility to explain why the radiologic examination is necessary, to answer patient questions, and to respond to any concerns about the nature of the examination. Poor communication between the doctor and the patient, the doctor and the radiographer, and/or the radiographer and the patient may result in a repeat examination or even in the wrong patient being radiographed. Communication then becomes an important factor in reducing unnecessary or excessive radiation exposure. Patients have the right to know about the examination; and if inadequately informed, they may have questions or fears regarding the nature, purpose, or even value of the examination. Patients who do not understand what is going to happen or what is expected may even be reluctant to cooperate.

What responsibility does the radiographer have in regard to explaining the radiographic examination to the patient? It is the radiographer's responsibility to give the patient clear, concise instructions and to communicate in such a way that patients understand what is expected of them in order to complete the examination. If at any time the patient refuses to undergo the examination, the radiographer should seek supervisory assistance and never insist that the patient submit to any procedure against his/her will.

One way to ensure that each patient is informed regarding his/her radiographic examination is to take adequate time to explain the procedure so that the patient understands. The radiographer should always answer patient questions within ethical limitations, and if asked a question that cannot be answered, the radiographer should seek supervisory assistance. Remember, patients have the right to be completely informed about their medical care and to have their questions answered.

Patient Preparation.   Radiation protection also extends to patient preparation. Many repeat examinations occur as a result of inadequate patient preparation. It is important to ask the patient to remove all radiopaque objects from the area to be radiographed, such as necklaces, zippers, hair pins, and even long, braided hair. Remember that a repeat examination results in a repeat or double-radiation exposure to the patient.

During patient preparation and initial introductions, it is also important to give instructions regarding breath and motion control.

If positioning or immobilization devices are to be used, explain to the patient why they are needed and how they will be used. Talk to the patient before, during, and after the examination and let the patient be of assistance whenever possible.

Careful attention to radiographic positioning also helps reduce the number of retake radiographs and thus reduces unnecessary radiation exposure. Radiographers should never attempt a radiographic procedure if they are uncertain as to the correct procedure. If in doubt or just inexperienced, the radiographer should *STOP* and *ASK FOR HELP*.

Primary-Beam Limitation

Primary-beam limitation means using a device such as an aperture diaphragm, cone, or collimator to limit the useful or primary radiation beam to the area of clinical interest, thereby decreasing the area of body tissue irradiated. This in turn reduces the amount of secondary scattered radiation and also limits unnecessary exposure to the nearby tissue. A beam restrictor, however, is only as effective as the operator who uses the device. Therefore, it is important that radiographers understand the basic operation of each type of beam restrictor and the operator's role in using the device.

The aperture diaphragm is a simple beam-limitation device consisting of a flat piece of lead with a hole in the middle, Figure 12-1. The size and shape of the hole determine the size and shape of the radiographic beam.

An aperture diaphragm is constructed so that it fits directly below the X-ray tube window. One disadvantage of an aperture diaphragm is that each is designed to be used with a specific film size at a given distance. Because of this feature, it is not easily adaptable to various film sizes or distances. The variable-aperture diaphragm device overcomes this disadvantage because it has a variable opening

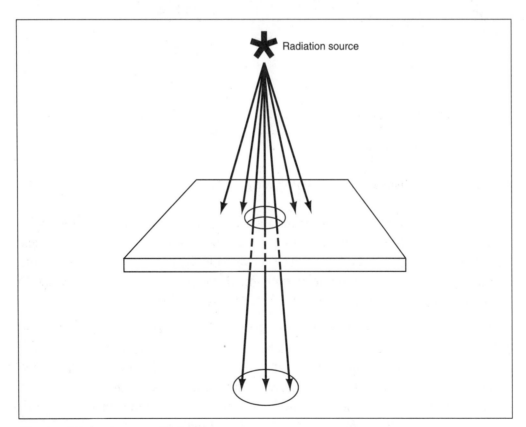

Figure 12-1 Aperture diaphragm

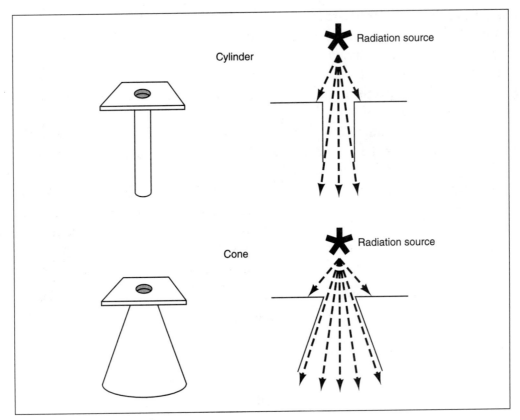

Figure 12-2   Beam-limitation devices

that can be adjusted for use with various film sizes and source-to-image distances.

Other simple beam-limitation devices are the cone (a circular metal tube with a flared end) and the cylinder (a long tube having the same diameter at base and tip), Figure 12-2. These devices—available in a variety of lengths and diameters—can be inserted and interchanged under the X-ray tube window to accommodate various film sizes and source-to-image distances.

Collimators.   A collimator, often referred to as a variable collimator, is an efficient beam-limitation device. Attached to the radiographic tube housing, the collimator looks like a square box with a clear plastic window. It contains two sets of adjustable lead shutters mounted at different levels, a light source, and a mirror to deflect the light source. The lead shutters can be adjusted so as to limit the primary radiation beam to the area of clinical interest, Figure 12-3.

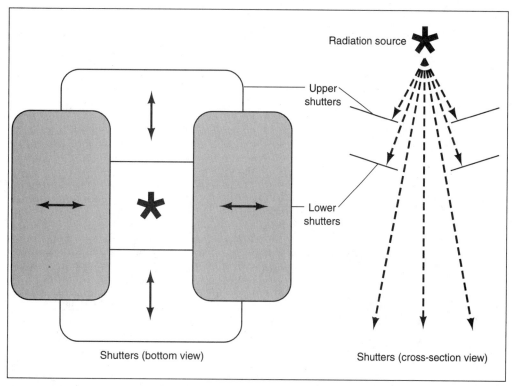

Radiation source

Upper shutters

Lower shutters

Shutters (bottom view)

Shutters (cross-section view)

Figure 12-3 Two views of shutters

Proper collimation of the primary radiation beam will result in an unexposed margin around the edge of the radiograph. Never allow the primary radiation beam to expose an area beyond the area of clinical interest. The examples in Figure 12-4 illustrate proper and improper collimation technique.

The collimator is equipped with a light source that simulates the radiation exposure area. The collimator light is used as a guide in positioning, alignment, central ray placement, and collimation. If the light source becomes misaligned with the actual area of radiation exposure, errors in positioning, alignment, central ray placement, or collimation may occur. Daily use, a bump, or jarring of the collimator housing may result in misalignment. The radiographer should include a collimator-light-source-accuracy check as part of a scheduled routine equipment-maintenance check. Whenever in doubt about the collimator-light-source accuracy, perform a light-source-accuracy check.

The efficiency of any beam-restricting device depends upon its regular and proper use by the radiographer. The positive beam limitation (PBL) system was

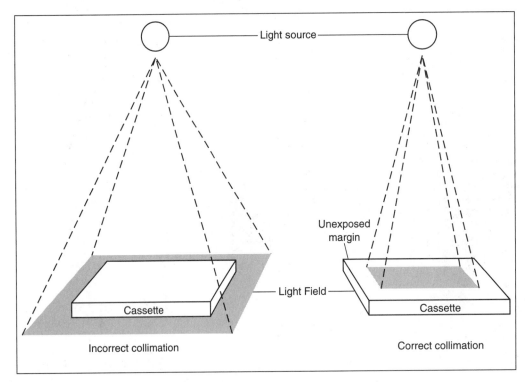

Figure 12-4   Proper use of collimation

designed in response to the concern about the operator forgetting to limit the beam. The PBL system actually restricts the primary beam to the film size used in the bucky tray. The PBL system consists of electronic sensors installed in the bucky tray holder. When a film holder is locked into the bucky tray, the electronic sensors transmit the film size information to the collimator, which automatically adjusts the primary beam to the size of the film holder, Figure 12-5.

An additional benefit of restricting the primary beam is improved radiographic quality. A properly collimated primary radiation beam produces less secondary scattered radiation, thus reducing possible film fog or increased film darkening.

Filtration.   Filtration of the primary radiation beam is another method used to protect the patient from unnecessary radiation exposure. Radiographic filters serve two major functions by removing low-energy, long-wavelength photons from the primary beam. These functions are to 1) protect the patients' skin and superficial tissue and 2) improve the quality of the radiation beam. By removing the longer wavelengths, the beam is more homogeneous in wavelength. This

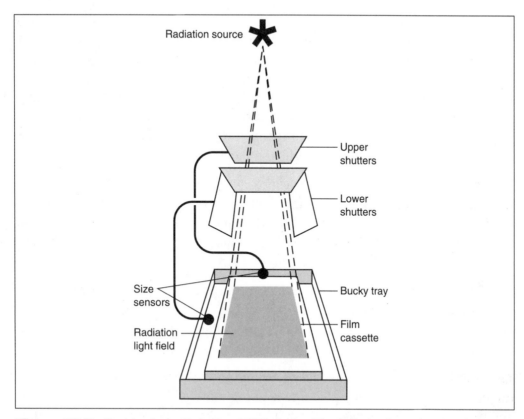

Radiation source

Upper
shutters

Lower
shutters

Size
sensors

Bucky tray

Radiation
light field

Film
cassette

Figure 12-5 Positive beam limitation (PBL) device. The radiation beam is properly limited from the source (tube) to the cassette.

filtering is referred to as attenuation of the beam. Ultimately, as primary radiation is restricted and filtered, there is less radiation to scatter.

There are two types of radiographic filtration: inherent filtration and added filtration. Inherent filtration consists of the tube's glass envelope, insulating oil, and the glass window. Inherent filtration is expressed in equivalent aluminum thickness and should be at least 0.5 mm of aluminum. Aluminum is the metal of choice because it effectively removes long wavelengths, is inexpensive, and is sturdy.

Added filtration is any filtration added to the existing inherent filtration. These filters, usually consisting of aluminum sheets, may be added outside the tube housing. The inherent filtration plus added filtration represent the required amount of total filtration. The amount of total radiographic-tube filtration is dependent upon the kilovoltage ranges of the equipment, e.g., 50–70 kVp = 1.5 mm aluminum; above 70 kVp = 2.5 mm aluminum.

Film Screen Combinations.   Patient radiation dose is affected by the choice of film-screen combination. The dose to the patient will be lessened when a high-speed film-screen combination is used. The speed of the imaging system describes the way in which the intensifying screen enhances the action of the X rays and the way the film responds. Use of a rare-earth imaging system rather than calcium tungstate screens will reduce the patient's radiation dose. This is possible since rare-earth screens are from two to ten times as fast as calcium tungstate screens and emit more light and therefore less initial X-ray exposure.

Grids.   The primary purpose of a grid, whether stationary or moving, is to minimize scattered radiation, which degrades the radiographic image. A grid is placed between the patient and the film and serves to improve radiographic image quality, thus contributing to the reduction of retake radiographs and therefore reducing additional radiation exposure to the patient.

Air-Gap Technique.   Air-gap technique may be used when a grid is needed but not available. A distance or "natural" air gap is introduced between the patient and the film holder. This distance allows the scattered photons emerging from the patient to diverge and never reach the film.

Gonadal Shielding.   Gonadal shielding protects the patients' gonads from direct primary exposure by placing shielding material between the X-ray beam and the patients' gonads. Gonadal shielding should be used in addition to primary beam restriction and never as a substitute for it.

Gonad shielding should be provided for all persons having reproductive potential, including adults of reproductive age and children. The anatomic location of the testes allows for adequate shielding while not obscuring needed clinical information. The ovaries, however, located near the vertebral spine, ureters, and small and large intestines, do not permit adequate shielding without obscuring a great deal of anatomy nearby.

The two kinds of gonadal shields are *shadow shields* and *contact shields*. Shadow shields are so named because of the shadow cast by the shields. These shields are suspended from the beam-limiting system. They can be positioned to hang over the patients' gonads and are positioned with the assistance of a light localizer. Contact shields may be flat, uncontoured, lead-impregnated material placed on or taped to the patient to cover the gonads, or they may be shaped and contoured to enclose the male reproductive organs, Figure 12-6.

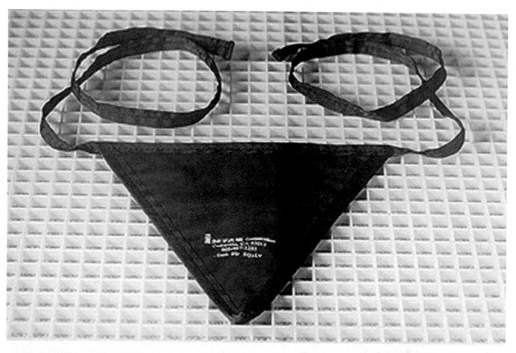

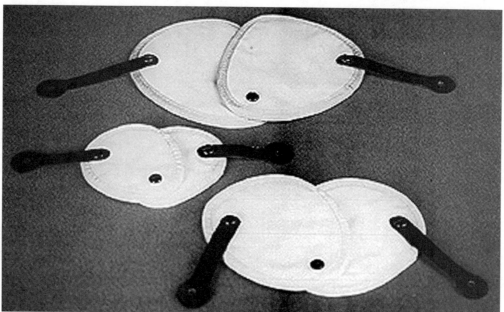

Figure 12-6   Examples of gonadal shields *(Courtesy of GE Medical Systems)*

Flat contact shields are most effective for anterior-posterior or posterior-anterior projections when the patient is recumbent. Flat contact shields can be easily used for male and female patients; whereas the shaped contact shield is designed exclusively for use with male patients.

Shaped contact shields are used with disposable supporters. The cup-shaped shield permits enclosure of the scrotum and penis and remains in place with the patient in an upright or recumbent position.

Gonadal shields should meet the following specifications based on the kVp range used:

0.25 mm lead equivalent for 100 kVp or less
0.5 mm lead equivalent for 100–150 kVp
1.0 mm lead equivalent for 150 kVp and above

The decision to use gonadal shielding must be considered with each individual patient's situation and the radiographic request. However, the following criteria provide guidelines for deciding when gonadal shielding should be used:

1. Use gonadal shielding on all patients who have a reasonable likelihood of reproducing.
2. Use gonadal shielding on all children.
3. Use gonadal shielding if the gonads lie within the primary beam or within 5 cm (2½ in) of the primary beam's edge.
4. Use gonadal shielding if the shielding will not obscure (cover) necessary diagnostic information on the radiograph.

Gonadal shields can develop cracks and pinpoint holes with constant use or if improperly stored. Gonadal shields should be stored flat without folds when not in use and should be regularly checked for cracks or pinpoint holes, which can allow radiation leaks to the patient.

Technical Factor Selection.   Selection of the correct combination of technical factors has a direct impact on the amount of radiation received by the patient. Table 12-4 lists technical factors and their roles in radiation protection.

PREGNANT PATIENT

Observing all radiation-protection guidelines is extremely important if the patient is pregnant or a pregnancy is suspected. It is important to remember that

TABLE 12-4 ▪ Technical Factors/Roles

FACTOR	EFFECT
Exposure selection of high kVp and low mAs	Reduces radiation dose
Proper film processing	Reduces repeat examinations
Use of a grid	Improves radiographic quality
Use of intensifying screen	Reduces amount of radiation exposure required
	Reduces patient radiation dose
Reduction of repeat examinations	Reduces radiation dose

it is the doctor's responsibility to evaluate the patient and to determine if the diagnostic benefits outweigh the risks associated with radiation exposure. The radiographer's responsibility is to avoid unnecessary radiation exposure and to produce diagnostic-quality radiographs while providing for patient comfort and safety. This can be accomplished by performing all recommended radiation-protection procedures and by providing the pregnant patient with a lead apron or shield placed over the uterus or totally surrounding the pelvis, Figure 12-7.

Radiation-protection procedures for the potentially pregnant patient conform to the ALARA concept. The use of the "ten day rule," which stated that pelvic or abdominal examinations of women of child-bearing age be done only in the first ten days following the onset of menstruation, is no longer used. The guideline to follow is that *all* radiographic procedures be performed in a manner to keep the radiation exposure as low as reasonably achievable.

Although the major responsibility for patient radiation-safety rests with the doctor and radiographer, the current trend in consumer awareness and involvement focuses some responsibility to the patient. This responsibility involves the patient being aware, asking questions about medical care, and adopting a personal philosophy of not requesting diagnostic radiographic procedures when alternative diagnostic measures are suggested by the attending physician. The United States Food and Drug Administration has responded to this new focus on consumer awareness by developing an X-ray record card similar to immunization record cards.

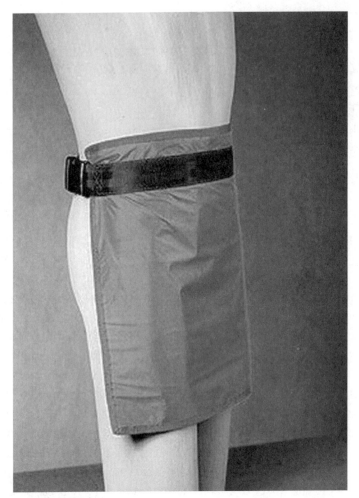

Figure 12-7   Patient protective apron *(Courtesy of GE Medical Systems)*

RADIATION-PROTECTION PROCEDURES FOR THE OPERATOR

Cardinal Principles

There are three cardinal principles of radiation protection: time, distance, and shielding (TDS), Figure 12-8. If used together, the principles of TDS can minimize radiation exposure to the patient and radiographer. These three cardinal principles were developed for nuclear-energy employees who have the potential to be exposed to high levels of radiation in their workplace. The radiographer, of

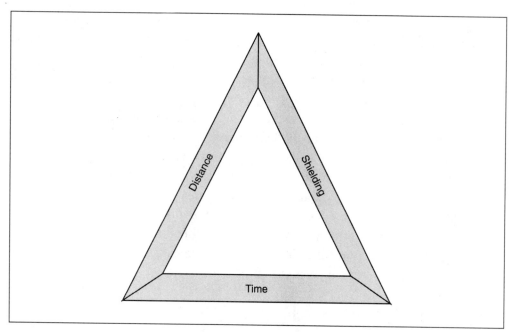

Figure 12-8   Three cardinal principles of radiation protection

course, is not expected to be employed in a high-level radiation area, such as a nuclear energy plant, but the cardinal principles have practical application to medical radiography.

Time.   Radiation exposure is proportional to the amount of time spent in the radiation. A five-minute exposure to radiation would result in a radiation dose five times as great as a one-minute exposure to radiation. This has several implications that can be related to the radiographer and the patient. The radiographer has a responsibility to:

1. Reduce the amount of time exposed to radiation. Do not stay in a radiography room during the exposure unless standing behind a protective barrier.
2. Reduce the amount of time that the patient is exposed to radiation. Reduce retake examinations and subsequently reduce time and radiation exposure.
3. Use a fast exposure-time factor whenever possible. A fast exposure time can reduce radiographic motion unsharpness due to patient movement.

Distance.   Distance between the radiographer and the radiation source is the most effective way to reduce radiation exposure and the most easily applied principle of radiation protection. The inverse square law which applies to point sources of radiation can be used to demonstrate the effect of distance on radiation intensity, Figure 12-9. Radiation from an X-ray tube is considered to be a point source. Radiation intensity from a point source varies inversely as the square of the distance from the source.

X rays are similar to light in that the further you move away from the source, the dimmer the light becomes or the less intense the X rays become. Figure 12-9 demonstrates that doubling the distance in an X-ray exposure will spread the radiation over four (4) times the original area size; therefore, the radiation will have only one-fourth its original intensity. Distance is a very important safety guideline because operator protection increases as the distance from the radiation source increases. For example, as the distance doubles from the radiation source, the radiographer gains four times more protection because the radiation intensity is decreased by one-fourth its original intensity.

In clinical situations where mobile radiographic equipment is used, special protection considerations apply. If structural or mobile protective shielding is

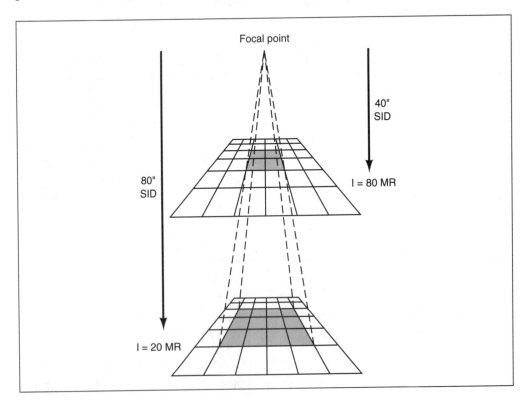

Figure 12-9   Inverse square law

not available, the radiographer should wear a protective lead apron and gloves. The exposure switch cord should be at least 6 feet (72 inches) long to permit the operator to gain maximum of a 72-inch distance from the radiation source (inverse square law application). The radiographer should also position his/her body at a right angle (90 degrees) to the object creating scatter radiation. Use of the cardinal principals of time, distance, and shielding should be applied to maximize radiation-protection measures to the operator and patient.

The distance principle as applied to patient protection means that every radiographic examination should be performed with the X-ray tube positioned at the proper SID from the patient or part being examined.

Shielding.   Shielding is the third cardinal principle of radiation protection. As X-ray photons travel through the air or through an absorber (such as living tissue), the quantity and energy of the X-ray photons decrease. The degree to which the quantity and energy of the X-ray photons is decreased depends upon several factors: 1) original quantity and energy of the X-ray beam; 2) type of absorber material; and 3) thickness of the absorber material. If X-ray photons travel through enough absorbing material, eventually their energy will be lost to the material and no X rays will emerge through to the other side.

Protective shields are usually constructed of lead or a concrete wall barrier. This serves as an absorber of the radiation and should be situated so that it intercepts the primary radiation and any radiation that has scattered.

The radiographer should stand behind a lead shield or wall barrier when making the radiographic exposure. The radiographer should not peek around the shield or wall to watch the patient but should watch the patient through the protective glass window installed in the shield or wall, Figure 12-10.

Structural Protective Shielding

When a radiography room is designed, a qualified medical physicist will survey the prospective room and determine the exact shielding requirements. Whether the prospective radiography room is already in existence or is part of a new construction, appropriate thickness of lead will be installed according to the medical physicist's specifications. The medical physicist will recommend and provide recommendations for primary and secondary protective barriers.

Primary Protective Shielding.   Primary protective shielding provides protection from the primary X-ray beam. For equipment capable of operating up to the 150 kVp range, protective primary shielding should consist of 1/16th inch lead

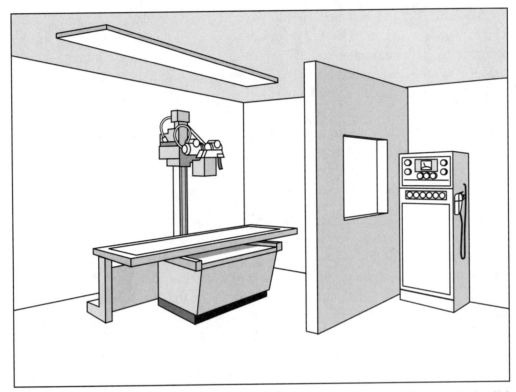

Figure 12-10   Arrangement of a control console of an X-ray machine with protective leaded wall and window *(Courtesy of GE Medical Systems)*

and be as high as 7 feet from the X-ray room floor. Primary protective shielding is located perpendicular to the primary X-ray beam.

Secondary Protective Shielding.   Secondary radiation occurs when the primary X-ray photons are deflected or re-directed by the object being irradiated. Radiation leakage around the X-ray tube and scatter radiation generated by the patient and other objects receiving radiation comprise secondary radiation. Secondary protective shielding should consist of $^1/_{32}$nd inch of lead, extend to the ceiling, and be located parallel to the primary beam. Secondary protective shielding barriers, such as the control console shield or structural barrier, often contain a window through which the operator can observe the patient. The window is required to contain 1.5 mm lead equivalent.

Protective Apparel

Protective apparel is used for the patient and radiographer whenever additional protection is desired or necessary. Protective apparel consists of lead-impregnated vinyl gloves and apron, Figure 12-11. When operating in the kVp range of 100, the lead gloves and apron should be at least 0.25 mm lead equivalency; however, lead aprons are typically lined with 0.5 mm lead or its equivalency.

Handle lead aprons, gloves, and gonad shields with care. Protective apparel should be properly stored when not in use to prevent cracks from developing in the lead. Do not store the items by folding since cracks could result from

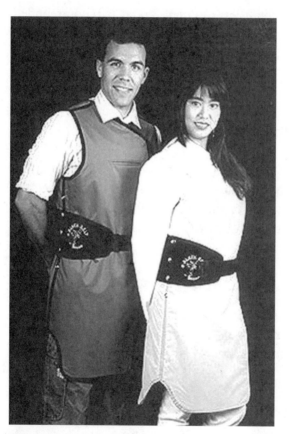
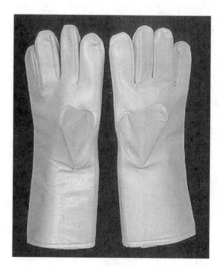

Figure 12-11 Use of lead apron and gloves for personal protection *(Courtesy of GE Medical Systems)*

the bending of the protective lead insert. Cracks could permit radiation to leak through.

The lead apron and gloves should be checked for cracks once every three months.

The Pregnant Radiographer

A radiographer who becomes pregnant while employed in that capacity should discuss her pregnancy with her supervisor and attending physician. These three persons should review together all radiation-protection guidelines. The dose equivalent is 5 mSv (0.5 rem) for the total period of the pregnancy and 0.5 mSv (0.05 rem) for any given month. Remember, the first trimester (first three months) is the most critical period of fetal development, and it is recommended that the pregnant radiographer receive as little radiation exposure as possible.

Optional protective measures that a pregnant radiographer may use include wearing a protective lead apron of at least 0.5 mm lead in addition to standing behind the protective barrier and wearing a "Baby" film badge. The "Baby" film badge may be worn in addition to the operator film badge. The badge worn near the hip or pelvic area should be labeled "Baby" so that a separate record can be maintained.

If a pregnant radiographer performs the usual recommended radiation safety procedures during all radiography examinations and uses the optional protective measures outlined, it is nearly impossible for the radiographer to be exposed to the fetal dose equivalent. Pregnancy does not justify a lay-off or termination of employment.

RADIATION DETECTION AND MONITORING

Accurate radiation detection and measurement is necessary if occupational exposure levels are to be kept below the maximum-permissible-dose levels. Personnel and area monitoring are the most commonly used procedures used to determine occupational exposure.

Personnel Monitoring Devices

Personnel monitoring provides important information regarding the amount of radiation exposure received by an operator. The information gathered from personnel monitoring must then be reviewed to determine if it is within the maximum-permissible-dose guidelines. After the review, corrective actions may be required to reduce or eliminate the radiation exposure. It should be recognized that personnel radiation monitoring is just that—a monitor that records the amount of radiation received and is an indication of the radiographer's working habits and working conditions. One should never assume one is safe just because monitoring is occurring. Nor should it be assumed that because no exposure has ever been recorded, no exposure has ever been or ever will be received. Also, personnel monitoring devices record only the exposure received in the area in which they are worn. The device should be attached to the front of the clothing so it records the radiation received by the radiographer's body trunk. During fluoroscopic procedures when the operator wears a protective lead apron, an additional monitoring device may be worn outside of the protective apron at the collar level to record exposure to the radiosensitive organs of the head, neck, and lens of the eye.

There are three basic kinds of personnel-radiation-monitoring devices: film badges, thermoluminescent dosimeters, and pocket ionization chambers. Usually, the nature of the occupation and the type of ionizing radiation will determine the choice of personnel monitoring device. A summary of personnel monitoring devices is presented in Table 12-5.

Film Badges.   Film badges are the most frequently used type of personnel monitoring device. They are economical and considered relatively accurate in recording low doses of radiation if instructions regarding care and use are followed.

A film badge consists of three parts: a film packet, metal filters, and a plastic holder with a clip attachment, Figure 12-12. The plastic holder is made of a low-atomic-number material so that low-energy radiation may reach the film packet. Metal filters of aluminum or copper are contained in the plastic holder and allow for measurement of the radiation energy reaching the film packet. After processing, the degree of film-darkening beneath the filters provides a basis for estimating the radiation exposure. A densitometer is used to measure film density and is then compared to the exposure value of a control film of similar density on a characteristic curve. In addition to the amount of radiation received, the information provided by film-badge films also includes: 1) direction of the radiation exposure (from front to back or from back to front) and 2) whether exposure was from excessive scattered radiation or a single primary beam exposure.

TABLE 12-5 ▪ Summary of Personnel Monitoring Devices

DEVICE	ADVANTAGES	DISADVANTAGES
Film Badge	▪ Economical, low-cost ▪ Durable container ▪ Permanent record of personnel exposure ▪ Detects both small and large exposures ▪ Filters allow determination regarding direction of exposure and cause of exposure (scatter/primary) ▪ Control badge provided ▪ Reliable with X-ray and gamma radiation and differentiates between	▪ Only effective if worn and cared for according to monitoring company directions ▪ Records exposure only in area where badge is worn ▪ Film packet can be fogged by excessive temperature or humidity
TLD Device	▪ Accurately records dose ▪ Not sensitive to excessive temperature or humidity ▪ May be worn up to three months	▪ Initial high cost ▪ No permanent record of readings ▪ Not effective if not worn ▪ Person performing readout must follow recommended procedures
Pocket Ionization Chamber	▪ Easy to wear ▪ Sensitive and accurately records dose ▪ Immediate readout in self-reading chambers	▪ Expensive ▪ No permanent record of readings ▪ Chamber should be read and recharged daily ▪ Not effective if not worn

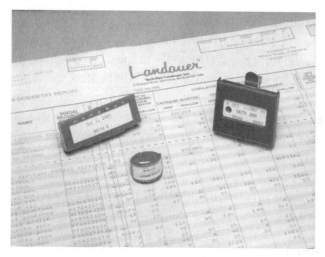

Figure 12-12 *(Left to right)* A typical film badge, thermoluminescent dosimeter ring, and collar badge. *(Courtesy of Tech/O Landauer, Inc.)*

The radiographic-film packet consists of radiation dosimetry film and is similar in size and shape to dental film. Enclosed in a light-free envelope, the radiographic film has sensitivity to doses ranging from 0.1 mSv (10 millirems) to 5 Sv (500 rems). The light-free envelope has a lead foil back that absorbs scatter radiation from behind the device.

Film-badge film packets must be returned to the monitoring company at specific intervals (usually once a month) for processing. The monitoring company provides a control film packet with each shipment of film packets. The control film packet serves as a control for comparing the worn film packets after they have been returned for processing. The control film packet must be stored in a radiation-free area within the medical facility.

Monitoring companies provide a written report containing the results for each film packet and the control packet. These film-badge reports should be reviewed by the facility's radiation safety officer or supervisor to determine compliance with effective-absorbed-dose-equivalents limits guidelines and corrective action taken as necessary. The badge reports should be permanently maintained with personnel records.

Although film badges have the advantage of being economical and not easily damaged if dropped, the disadvantages must be considered. The film packet is sensitive to extreme temperature and humidity levels and is not accurate over long periods of recording time, generally not longer than one month.

Thermoluminescent Dosimeters.   A thermoluminescent dosimeter (TLD) badge is similar in appearance to the film badge; however, it contains a different type of monitoring system. Special crystals in the TLD undergo physical property changes when struck by ionizing radiation. When heated, the crystals emit energy in the form of visible light, equal to the amount of radiation exposure absorbed. A TLD analyzer is then used to heat and measure the amount of radiation received. TLD monitoring devices have several advantages that film badges do not have. They give more accurate recording of low radiation doses; they are less sensitive to extreme temperatures or humidity; and they can be used for up to three months. Disadvantages include initial high cost and no permanent record of the radiation reading since the readout process destroys the stored information.

Pocket Ionization Chambers.   The most sensitive, yet infrequently used, personnel monitoring device in diagnostic radiology is the pocket ionization chamber. The pocket dosimeter resembles a fountain pen and contains an ionization chamber, which may be either a self-reading type or a non-self-reading chamber (which requires the use of a special electrometer accessory for a readout).

One advantage of the pocket ionization chamber is that the self-reading type can provide an immediate exposure readout. This is an important and critical feature often required by those who work in high-radiation-exposure occupations. These chambers are expensive and require careful attention to the manufacturer's directions during the readout.

Survey Instruments for Area Monitoring

Radiation survey instruments are used to detect the presence or absence of radiation in a particular area. Generally, radiographers will not be required to use survey instruments to determine radiation exposure; however, it is important to recognize the function of these instruments. The Geiger-Müller (G-M) detector, ionization chamber-type survey meter, and the proportional counter are gas-filled radiation survey instruments used to detect radiation and its exposure quantity. The Victoreen condenser R-meter used to calibrate radiography equipment is also a gas-filled ionization chamber. Survey instruments are commonly used by radiation physicists, equipment inspectors, X-ray service staff, and others who are employed in nuclear occupations where environmental radiation exposure may occur.

REVIEW QUESTIONS ──────────────────────────

1. The main goal of all radiation protection procedures
   a) is to reduce radiation exposure to zero
   b) allows exposures up to the maximal limits
   c) is to limit only nonoccupational exposures
   d) is to keep all radiation exposures as low as reasonably achievable

2. The annual effective-absorbed-dose-equivalent limits for whole-body occupational exposure is
   a) 5 mSv (0.5 rem)
   b) 50 mSv (5 rem)
   c) 150 mSv (15 rem)
   d) 500 mSv (50 rem)

3. The annual effective-absorbed-dose-equivalent limits for embryo-fetus exposure to term is
   a) 5 mSv (0.5 rem)
   b) 50 mSv (5 rem)
   c) 150 mSv (15 rem)
   d) 500 mSv (50 rem)

4. The annual effective-absorbed-dose-equivalent limits for infrequent, non-occupational exposure is
   a) 5 mSv (0.5 rem)
   b) 50 mSv (5 rem)
   c) 150 mSv (15 rem)
   d) 500 mSv (50 rem)

5. The cumulative lifetime exposure for a fifty-year-old radiation worker is
   a) 5 mSv (0.5 rem)
   b) 50 mSv (5 rem)
   c) 150 mSv (15 rem)
   d) 500 mSv (50 rem)

6. Which of the following areas can contribute to reducing patient radiation exposure?
    1. patient communication
    2. patient preparation
    3. primary beam limitation
        a) 1 and 2
        b) 1 and 3
        c) 2 and 3
        d) 1, 2, and 3

7. Methods of limiting the primary beam include
    1. aperture diaphragm
    2. cone
    3. collimator
        a) 1 and 2
        b) 1 and 3
        c) 2 and 3
        d) 1, 2, and 3

8. Which of the following is true?
    1. Increasing distance increases radiation exposure.
    2. Decreasing exposure time decreases radiation exposure.
    3. Increasing shielding decreases radiation exposure.
        a) 1 and 2
        b) 1 and 3
        c) 2 and 3
        d) 1, 2, and 3

9. Some advantages of using a film badge for personnel monitoring include
    1. low cost
    2. reliability
    3. not sensitive to excessive humidity or temperature
        a) 1 and 2
        b) 1 and 3
        c) 2 and 3
        d) 1, 2, and 3

10. Some advantages of using a thermoluminescent dosimeter (TLD) for personnel monitoring include
    1. low cost
    2. accuracy
    3. not sensitive to excessive humidity or temperature
       a) 1 and 2
       b) 1 and 3
       c) 2 and 3
       d) 1, 2, and 3

11. The most important role of primary beam filtration is to reduce
    a) radiation scatter
    b) X-ray technique
    c) damage to patient's skin and superficial tissue
    d) need to collimate

12. The main goal of all radiation protection activities is to conduct
    a) reciprocity
    b) ALARA
    c) TDS
    d) LET

13. All of the following will contribute to reducing patient radiation exposure, **EXCEPT**
    a) good verbal communication
    b) limiting the primary beam
    c) retake examinations
    d) gonadal shielding

14. Select the example which illustrates the inverse square law.
    a) as the distance from the radiation source increases, the radiation exposure decreases
    b) as the distance from the radiation source decreases, the radiation exposure decreases
    c) as the distance from the radiation source decreases, the intensity of radiation remains the same
    d) none of the above

BIBLIOGRAPHY

Bushong, Stewart C. *Radiologic Science for Technologists: Physics, Biology, and Protection*, 6th edition, St. Louis, MO: Mosby-Year Book, 1997.

National Council on Radiation Protection and Measurements (NCRP) Report #54, *Medical Exposure of Pregnant and Potentially Pregnant Women*, Washington, DC: NCRP Publications, 1977.

National Council on Radiation Protection and Measurements (NCRP) Report #91, *Recommendations on Limits for Exposure to Ionizing Radiation*, Bethesda, MD: NCRP Publications, 1987.

Statkiewicz-Sherer, Mary Alice, Paul J. Visconti, and E. Russell Ritenour. *Radiation Protection in Medical Radiography*, 3rd edition, St. Louis, MO: Mosby-Year Book, 1997.

Glossary

Absorbed dose   the amount of radiation energy absorbed in tissue; measured in greys

Acute dose   the amount of radiation received in a single exposure

ALARA concept   as low as reasonably achievable; the idea that radiation exposures be kept as low as possible

Alpha particle   a product of radioactive decay composed of two protons and two neutrons; a helium nucleus

Ampere   the S.I. base unit of electrical current; also expressed as 1 coulomb/second

Amplitude   the fluctuation of a wave above or below the normal non-perturbed state

Anion   a negatively charged particle

Anode   the positively charged side of an electrical circuit; the target side of an X-ray tube

Aperture diaphragm   an X-ray beam restrictor consisting of a lead sheet with a hole

Apnea   cessation of breathing

Apparent focal spot   the size of the projected X-ray tube focal spot

Area   the amount of enclosed space; height times width; measured in cm^2

Asymptomatic   without symptoms of disease or illness

Atom   the smallest particle that an element can be reduced to while still maintaining its chemical identity

Atomic mass number   the number of protons and neutrons in a nucleus

Atomic number   the number of protons in a nucleus

Automatic exposure control (AEC)   X-ray exposure timing determined by a radiation sensitive detector

Autonomy   freedom to govern one's self or self-governance

Autotransformer   a transformer consisting of two windings on a single core; used in x-ray machines to change the line voltage

Axilla   the region under the shoulder, commonly referred to as the armpit

Background radiation   the normal amount of radiation exposure expected from unavoidable natural and artificial sources

Beam restriction   control of the field size of an x-ray beam

Becquerel   the S.I. of radioactivity; equal to one disintegration per second

Beneficience   in health care, a duty to others to provide or improve conditions that promote physical and emotional well-being

Beta particle   a product of radioactive decay physically identical to an electron

Biomedical ethics   ethics applied to the knowledge of modern medical technologies

Body language   nonverbal indicators of communication, e.g., smiling, frowning, clenched fists

Calcium tungstate   a material developed by Thomas A. Edison and used in intensifying screens

Cassette   a rigid holder that contains intensifying screens; used to hold film

Cathode   the negatively charged side of an electrical circuit; the side of an X-ray tube where electrons are produced

Cation   a positively charged particle

Cheyne-Stokes   abnormal breathing in which apnea (cessation of breathing) occurs from 10–60 seconds

Circuit breaker   a device used to quickly shut down an electrical circuit in case of overload

Classical scatter   an interaction of an X-ray photon with an atom that results in a change of direction of the photon with no loss of energy

Collimator   an adjustable X-ray beam restrictor

Compound   a substance composed of like molecules

Compton effect   an interaction of an x-ray photon with an atom that results in scattered, lower energy photon and an electron

Conductor   a material that carries electricity easily

Cone   a conical shaped X-ray beam restrictor

Confidentiality   a patient's legal and ethical right to privacy

Consumer-Patient Radiation Safety Act   enacted in 1981, it gives Congress the power to protect consumers and patients from unnecessary or excessive radiation exposure

Contact shield   a protective radiation shield that is in physical contact with the patient

Continuing education unit (CEU)   a unit of education usually designed to provide a review or update of technical information to credentialed individuals

Contrast differences seen between body organs and tissue thicknesses; controlled by kVp

Coulomb the S.I. unit of electrical charge; one A · s

Curie the obsolete unit of radioactivity; equal to 3.7×10^{10} disintegrations per second

Current the flow of electrons in an electrical circuit

Density overall blackness of the radiographic image; controlled by mAs

Diastolic the phase of the cardiac cycle in which the heart muscle is at rest

Diode an electrical device that allows the flow of electricity in one direction only

Distortion variation from normal shape; a misshapen radiographic image

DNA deoxyribonucleic acid; the biomolecule that carries genetic information

Dose rate the amount of radiation delivered per unit time; can be measured in sieverts per minute

Dyspnea difficult or labored breathing

Effective dose equivalent the total radiation exposure of a human

Effective focal spot the size of the focal spot that is perceived on the film

Electric potential the ability of electricity to do work; measured in volts

Electricity the presence or movement of charged particles

Electrification imparting a charge to objects

Electrodynamics the movement of electrical charge

Electromagnetic radiation radiation consisting of an electrical component and a magnetic component; described in terms of energy, wavelength, and frequency

Electron a negatively charged fundamental particle found in atomic orbitals

Electron binding energy the amount of energy holding an electron in its orbital

Electrostatics attraction or repulsion due to electrical charge

Element a chemically distinguishable substance consisting of only one kind of atom

Empathy the ability to understand another's situation, such as fear, pain, anger, without actually having the emotion

Energy the ability to do work; usually divided into kinetic energy, the energy of motion, and potential energy, the energy of position; measured in joules

Ethics the philosophical study of human behavior or conduct

Febrile   having elevated body temperature; feverish

Filament   the heated wire in the cathode of an X-ray tube where electrons are produced

Filament current   the amount of electrical current flowing through the filament of an X-ray tube; measured in amperes

Film badge   a personnel radiation monitor that measures radiation exposure by use of film

Film fog   "undesirable" density (film darkening); obscures image details

Filter   a metal device used to attenuate X rays

Filtration   the use of a filter to attenuate X rays

Fluorescence   a type of luminescence or "lighting up" that occurs when certain phosphors (calcium tungstate) absorb radiation

Focal spot (FS)   the region of the X-ray tube target where the electron beam is focused

Focusing cup   the metal cup surrounding the filament in an X-ray tube that focuses the electron beam in the X-ray tube

Fomite   an object that has been contaminated with a pathogen and serves to spread disease

Fractionation   an X-ray exposure in multiple doses repeated over a period of time

Frequency   the repetition rate of electromagnetic radiation; measured in hertz

Full-wave rectification   a type of rectification that utilizes both halves of the AC voltage pulse

Gamma rays   high-energy electromagnetic radiation resulting from radioactive decay of a nucleus

Genetic effect   the ability of ionizing radiations to damage reproductive cells

Geometric factors   factors of distance and positioning that affect the radiographic quality

Gonadal shield   a radiation shield used to protect the reproductive organs

Gray   the S.I. unit of radiation absorbed dose; also expressed as joules per kilogram

Grid   a radiographic accessory constructed with lead strips to reduce the amount of scattered radiation from a given exposure reaching the image receptor (IR)

Half-value layer (HVL)   the amount of material needed to attenuate a radiation beam by 50%

Half-wave rectification   a type of rectification that utilizes only one half of the AC voltage pulse

Heat unit (HU)   a measure of the heat accumulated in the anode of an X-ray tube due to self-absorption in the anode

Heel effect   diminished X-ray intensity at the anode end of an X-ray tube due to self-absorption in the anode

Hertz   the S.I. unit of frequency; expressed as 1/s

High voltage transformer   the transformer in an X-ray machine circuit that steps up the voltage prior to use in the X-ray tube

Hypertension   an elevation in blood pressure that is influenced by conditions, diseases, emotional, and environmental stress

Hyperventilation   increased respiratory rate or breathing that is deeper than normal

Hypotension   a decrease in blood pressure

Illuminator (viewbox)   a metal framework housing fluorescent tubes that emit light of standard daylight color and intensity

Image shape   the true shape of the anatomy projected onto the image receptor so that there is no distortion or magnification

Impulse timer   an X-ray exposure timer that is energized to various time intervals

Inertia   the tendency of a moving body to remain in motion or a stationary body to remain at rest

Informed consent   an individual's right to disclosure of all information related to a medical procedure or treatment to assure the person's full understanding for voluntary consent to accept medical care

Intensifying screens   screens composed of fluorescent phosphors

International System of Units (SI Units)   the approved system of measurement based on the meter, second, kilogram, ampere; also called S.I. units

Ion   an electrically charged particle

Ion pair   the free electron and charged atom resulting from the ionization of an atom

Ionization   the imparting of charge to an atom by the removal or addition of an electron

Ionization chamber   a device used to measure the quantity of ionization caused by radiation

Ionizing radiation   electromagnetic or particulate radiation that imparts charge to atoms (X-rays)

Isotopes   a nuclear arrangement with differing neutron numbers and the same atomic numbers

Justice   the balancing and fair distribution of medical care, facilities, and resources for society

Kilogram   the S.I. base unit of mass

Kilovolt   thousands of volts; the unit used to measure the energy of an X-ray beam

Kilovolt peak (kVp)   the maximum voltage in an electrical voltage pulse

Kilovolt peak meter   the device that measures the energy of an X-ray beam

Law of Bergonié and Tribondeau   the relation of radiation sensitivity to mitotic state and differentiation

Law of Conservation of Energy   the physical principle that energy can neither be created nor destroyed

Length   the spatial dimension of an object; measured in meters

Limited radiographer   a multi-skilled person dedicated to assisting in many aspects of medical care including basic radiography tasks under the supervision of a licensed practitioner of the healing arts

Line focus principle   the effect whereby the apparent focal spot is smaller than the actual focal spot of an X-ray tube

Linear energy transfer (LET)   the loss of energy to matter by radiation; measured in keV

Magnetism   the ability of certain materials to attract iron and other metals

Magnification   enlargement of the size of the actual anatomical part

Mass   the quantity of material in an object; measured in kilograms

mAs timer   an X-ray machine timer that terminates the exposure when a specific mAs is attained

Matter   the substance of an object; composed of atoms

Maximum permissible dose (MPD)   the maximum amount of radiation allowed under radiation safety standards; defined for the whole body, body parts, and calendar periods. MPD has been replaced by effective-absorbed-dose-equivalent limits

Meter   the S.I. base unit of length

Microorganisms   extremely small organisms: bacteria, fungi, protozoa, rickettsiae, and viruses

Milliammeter   the instrument used to measure X-ray tube current

Milliamperage (mA)   the unit of X-ray tube current

Milliamperage-seconds (mAs)   the product of X-ray tube current and exposure time; a measure of X-ray quantity

Molecule   chemical combinations of atoms into substances

Momentum   the product of mass and velocity

Motion   the property of movement

Negligible individual risk level (NIRL)   a level of risk that can be dismissed; the risk associated with an annual effective dose equivalent of 0.01 mSv

Neutron   an uncharged fundamental particle found in the nucleus of an atom

Nonmaleficience   in the health professions, to prevent harm or to cause no harm to another person

Nonpathogenic microorganisms   microscopic organisms that are not harmful

Nosocomial infection   opportunist infections; a group of pathogenic microorganisms that are common in medical settings

Nuclear energy   energy produced by fission or fusion of an atomic nucleus

Nucleus   1) the center of an atom containing neutrons and protons; 2) the portion of a cell containing the DNA

Object image distance (OID)   distance between the part being examined and the image receptor

Ohm   the S.I. unit of electrical resistance

Ohm's law   the physical principle which states that voltage is the product of current and resistance

Orbital   the preferred energy level in an atom for an electron

Overexposure   too much exposure of the film; usually too much density

Particulate radiation   ionizing radiation consisting of physical particles such as electrons or neutrons

Passbox   a light-tight passageway between the darkroom and outside areas. Allows passage to darkroom while preventing light from entering

Pathogenic organisms   microscopic organisms that are harmful and capable of causing disease

Penumbra   geometric blur (fuzziness) of the anatomical part being examined in the radiographic image

Philosophy   learning related to a search for truth and a general understanding of values and reality

Photoelectric effect   an interaction of an X-ray photon with an atom that results in the absorption of the X-ray and the emission of an electron

Photographic effect (PE)   effect of radiation or light on the emulsion of the film; quality of the image

Photographic factors   factors that control the optical properties of the image; density and contrast

Photons   the massless particles that convey electromagnetic force; X rays and light

Positive beam limitation (PBL)   a collimation device that automatically limits an X-ray beam according to the size of the image receptor

Potential difference   the difference in voltage in an electrical circuit

Power   the amount of work done per unit time; measured in watts

Primary circuit   the part of an X-ray machine circuit on the input side of the high voltage transformer

Professional   a highly skilled person; a person trained in the liberal arts or sciences and also possessing advanced education and training

Professional ethics   in the health related professions, standards of conduct that relate to duties and obligations of health care practitioners

Proton   a positively charged fundamental particle found in the nucleus of an atom

Protraction   a radiation exposure that occurs over a prolonged period of time

Rad   the obsolete unit of radiation absorbed dose

Radiation   electromagnetic waves or particular matter emitted as a result of electronic or atomic transitions

Radioactive decay (disintegration)   the release of radiation by an unstable nucleus

Radiographic artifact   areas of increased (+) or decreased (−) density on radiographs that represent no diagnostic information

Radiologic technologist   a person who has completed an approved educational program and passed an examination administered by the American Registry of Radiology Technologists

Radiosensitivity   the measure of the response of a biological organism to radiation

Rare-earth intensifying screens   screens composed of elements that belong to Group III in the periodic table of elements and have atomic numbers between 57 and 71

Reciprocity   law that states that response of film to radiation of a given intensity will remain unchanged if the milliamperage and time factors are equal

Rectifier   an electrical device that allows the flow of electricity in one direction only

Relative biologic effectiveness (RBE)   a measure of the biological effects of different types of radiations; the ratio of the effect of a standard radiation to a test radiation

Rem   Roentgen equivalent man; the obsolete unit of dose equivalent

Remnant radiation   now referred to as Exit Radiation Beam

Resistance   the property of a material that impedes the flow of electricity; measured in ohms

Resolution   ability of an imaging system of screens and films to produce and record the image of a part of human anatomy

Roentgen, Wilhelm Conrad   discovered X rays in 1895

Safelight illumination   incandescent lamps with a colored filter which allows light to be transmitted in the darkroom without fogging the film

Scattered radiation   the secondary radiation produced as a result of interactions of the primary radiation beam with atoms

Screen lag (afterglow)   phosphorescence or the presence of light or "glow" emitted by phosphors in an intensifying screen after the X-ray exposure has ceased

Second   the S.I. base unit of time

Secondary circuit   the part of an X-ray machine circuit on the output side of the high voltage transformer

Secondary radiation   electrons and scattered X-rays produced by X-ray interactions with atoms

Sensitometry   study of how radiographic film responds to radiation exposure photographically and to processing conditions chemically

Shadow shield   a radiation shield held or suspended above the patient

Sievert   the S.I. unit of dose equivalent; also expressed as one joule per kilogram

Silver halide crystals   active ingredient of the radiographic film emulsion

Silver recovery   a chemical or electrolytic process used to remove silver from radiographic fixer solution

Somatic effect   effect of radiation on the human body other than the gonads; responsible for cancer and cataracts

Source-to-image distance (SID)   distance from the tube (focal spot) to the image receptor

Step-down transformer   a transformer that reduces voltage

Step-up transformer   a transformer that increases voltage

Sympathy   acknowledgment of another person's grief, hurt, or loss

Symptomatic   having signs of disease or illness

Systolic   the phase of the cardiac cycle in which the heart muscle contracts

Target   1) the portion of an anode struck by the electron beam; 2) a radiation-sensitive cellular component

Target theory   the theory which states that there are one or two critical targets for radiation damage in a cell

Temperature   the amount of thermal kinetic energy in an object; measured in degrees celsius

Thermionic emission   the production of electrons by the heating of the X-ray tube filament

Thermoluminescent dosimeter   a personnel radiation monitoring device, which, when heated, produces light proportional to the radiation exposure

Time   the period when something occurs; measured in seconds or milliseconds

Transformer   an electrical device that increases the electrical voltage of a circuit

Tube current   the quantity of electrons flowing from the cathode to the anode; measured in mA

Tube rating charts   charts that identify safe combinations of X-ray tube operating kVp, mA, and exposure time relative to other characteristics of the unit and tube

Umbra   sharply (geometrically) defined edges of the anatomical part examined in the radiographic image

Underexposure   radiographic image that is too light; usually not enough density

Vector   an infected insect or animal that passes disease through a bite, e.g., ticks, fleas, lice

Velocity   the rate of motion of an object; measured in meters per second

Volt   the S.I. unit of electrical potential difference

Voltage compensator   a device in an X-ray machine circuit that corrects for fluctuations in line voltage

Volume   the amount of space contained in an object; measured in m^3

Watt   the S.I. unit of power; also expressed as joules per second

Wave   a periodic disturbance in a substance

Wavelength   the distance between two similar portions of a wave

Work   the expenditure of energy

X ray   a high energy, high frequency, short wavelength electromagnetic radiation

1997 CURRENTLY RECOGNIZED STANDARDIZATION OF TERMINOLOGY, ABBREVIATIONS, AND FORMATS

Absorbed dose   this unit is the rad and refers to the energy absorbed per unit of mass of radiated material

Accumulated dose 5(N-18)   this formula is obsolete due to changes enacted by the National Council on Radiation Protection (NCRP)

Anode/film distance   this is replaced by source to image distance (SID)

Automatic exposure control   replaces the term phototiming

Automatic positive beam limitation   this is replaced by automatic collimation

Blur   replaces the term recorded detail; describes the effect of patient motion on the radiograph; motion and blur are synonymous

Caldwell   refers to the term PA (Caldwell) projection

Contrast   radiographic contrast is defined as the visible differences between any two areas of radiographic density

Definition   term used is recorded detail

Distortion   the misrepresentation of the size or shape of a structure recorded in the radiographic image

Dose equivalent   unit is the rem and defined as absorbed dose multiplied by a quality factor that accounts for the difference in biological effectiveness of different types of radiation.

Dose equivalent limits   unit is used to refer to radiation exposure limits for radiation workers; replaces the term maximum permissible dose (MPD)

Entrance skin exposure   used in place of skin exposure

Exposure   unit of amount of exposure and is the Roentgen®

Exposure factors   refers to mA, kVp, time, and distance (SID)

Exposure latitude   the range of exposure factors that will produce a diagnostic radiograph

Film   refers to unexposed film; otherwise the term radiograph is used to refer to exposed film

Film contrast   the ability of the film emulsion to react to radiation and to record a particular range of densities

Film latitude   the ability of film to record a long range of density levels on the radiograph

Film latitude and film contrast   these two factors are dependent upon the sensitometric properties of the film and the processing conditions; they are directly determined from the characteristic H and D curve

Focal film distance (FFD)   replaced by SID

Grid radius   term used in grid focusing distance

Grid technique conversion factors   a variation in many textbooks exist to the answers are given in ranges

Lead glove thickness   .25 millimeters per NCRP report #102

Long scale contrast   means that the visual differences is slight but there are numerous densities

Loss of recorded detail   may also be called unsharpness or poor recorded detail and may be caused by patient motion or the use of a large focal spot

Object-film distance or OFD   replaced by OID

Position (radiographic position) used to describe a specific body part position, such as supine or prone. Refers to the patient's physical position

Projection refers to the path of the central ray

Radiograph film that has been exposed

Recorded detail sharpness of the structural lines as recorded in the radiographic image

Remnant radiation replaced by exit radiation or image forming radiation; refers to both the primary and secondary radiation; the primary radiation being responsible for the film darkening and the secondary radiation resulting in the latent image

Rhese used in the parietoorbital oblique (Rhese) projection

Scale of contrast the number of densities or shades of gray visible on the radiograph; selection of kilovoltage and subject contrast controls the scale of contrast produced

Screen speed a term used to express the screen system rather than names

Sharpness replaced by the term recorded detail

Sharpness of detail replaced by the term recorded detail

Short-scale contrast when there are abrupt differences in the densities present on the radiograph and the total number of densities is reduced.

SI units Sieverts, Grays, Becquerels are not used on the ARRT examination

Size distortion (magnification) enlargement of the recorded image when compared with the actual size of the structure

Shape distortion the structure will be elongated or foreshortened; a misrepresentation of the shape of the structure when compared with the actual shape of the structure

Stenvers used to refer to the posterior projection (Stenvers)

Subject contrast contrast resulting from the amount of radiation transmitted by a particular body part as a result of the differential absorption characteristics of the tissues and structures of the part

View refers to the body part as seen by the image recording media

Wavelength used when comparing one different forms

Appendix

TASKS

TASK 2-1

Using "I" Messages

Objective: To recognize and practice using common "I" messages.

Directions: Review the "I" message information, then write your "I" message in the practice activity.

Review Information Using "I" messages is effective when giving criticism, explaining a problem, making a suggestion, or expressing an opinion. "I" messages don't make others feel offended or put them in a defensive position. There are two parts to the "I" message. The *first part* describes your feelings without blaming anyone else for the way you feel.

"YOU" Message (blames others)	"I" Message (first part)
1. "You really make me mad."	1. "I'm feeling upset about this."
2. "You sure are disorganized."	2. "I like to have things well-organized."
3. "You're always interrupting."	3. "Maybe I'm talking too much."
4. "You don't understand."	4. _____
5. "You're walking too fast."	5. _____
6. "You're confusing me."	6. _____
7. "Your smoking bothers me."	7. _____

The *second part* of the "I" message describes how you would like to feel or how you would like the situation to be changed.

"I" Message (describes your feelings)	"I" Message (describes how you would like things to change)
1. "I'm having some difficulty following you."	1. "Could we go back to the first part of your story?"
2. "Although I don't agree, I hear your point of view."	2. "I'd like us to understand each other better."
3. "I'm concerned about the image of our office."	3. "I'm asking everyone to give special attention to personal appearance."

Practice Activities

1. The office staff is having a meeting to decide on a better supply inventory system. Judith insists that she knows the best way and will not give anyone else a chance to talk.

   "YOU" Message: "You're monopolizing the conversation."

   "I" Message, first part: "I appreciate your good ideas."

   "I" Message, second part: "I'd also like to hear some other opinion."

2. Several staff members are eating lunch in the office conference room. In a joking mood, they start to tease you about being the office supervisor's favorite. If your coworkers have a real problem over this, you would like to discuss it.

   "YOU" Message: "If you worked as hard as I do, you might get noticed too."

   "I" Message, first part: _____

   "I" Message, second part: _____

3. You have just started a new job. The supervisor keeps watching everything you do. You would like to be able to work more on your own.

   "YOU" Message: "You're making me nervous."

   "I" Message, first part: _____

   "I" Message, second part: _____

4. Rita collects the money for the coffee fund at work. Everyone is supposed to contribute, and you are the only one who does not drink coffee.

   "YOU" Message: "Rita, you're being unfair. You're the ones who drink the coffee."

   "I" Message, first part: _____

   "I" Message, second part: _____

5. You have noticed that patients often have to wait at the reception area while the receptionist makes appointments. Mrs. Bruce, your supervisor, walks by and you stop to tell her about it.

   "YOU" Message: "Mrs. Bruce, you really need to do something about these long lines."

   "I" Message, first part: _____

   "I" Message, second part: _____

TASK 2-2

Using Paraphrasing*

Objective: To recognize and practice using common paraphrasing techniques.

Directions: Review the paraphrasing examples. read the example statements, then complete the student self-check activity. Write your paraphrasing response.

Review Information Paraphrasing means repeating what a person has said to you, but using slightly different words. Paraphrasing a statement helps you determine whether you understood the message as it was intended. Review the example statements.

<table>
<tr><td align="center">**Example Statements**</td><td align="center">**Paraphrasing Examples**</td></tr>
<tr><td>

Patient to Radiographer:
"You know, I took a hard fall and my knee hurts more than the ankle you are X-raying."
</td><td>

Radiographer to Patient:
"*Are you saying* that your knee hurts as much as your ankle?"
</td></tr>
<tr><td>

Worker to Coworker:
"I want to go to my grandmother's birthday party next Saturday, but I'm afraid to ask for the day off."
</td><td>

Coworker to Worker:
"You sound anxious about asking the supervisor to have the day off."
</td></tr>
<tr><td>

Worker to Coworker:
"The new sick leave policy is really unfair."
</td><td>

Coworker to Worker:
_____
_____
_____
</td></tr>
<tr><td>

Patient to Radiographer:
"I'm really dreading the thought of having this chest X ray."
</td><td>

Radiographer to Patient:
_____
_____
_____
</td></tr>
<tr><td>

Patient to Account Clerk:
"This charge for a chest X ray seems really too high compared to the time it took the girl to take it."
</td><td>

Account Clerk to Patient:
_____
_____
_____
</td></tr>
<tr><td>

Patient to Radiographer:
"Now I'm going to tell you my old bones hurt and I can't just jump up on that cold table."
</td><td>

Radiographer to Patient:
_____
_____
_____
</td></tr>
</table>

*Adapted from M. M. Brewner, W. C. McMahon, and M. P. Roche. *Job Survival Skills*. New York: Educational Designs, Inc., 1984, p. 65.

TASK 2-3

Using Listening Techniques*

Objective: To recognize personal listening habits.

Directions: Rate your listening habits on the scale below by circling one of the numbers (1–5) after each item.

	Usually	Often	Sometimes	Not Usually	Hardly Ever
1. After only a short period of listening, I start thinking about what I'm going to say next.	1	2	3	4	5
2. If I don't like the person, I don't really listen to what she/he is saying.	1	2	3	4	5
3. I interrupt others before they are finished talking.	1	2	3	4	5
4. I fake attention.	1	2	3	4	5
5. I talk most about myself.	1	2	3	4	5
6. I ask questions.	5	4	3	2	1
7. I give other people a chance to talk.	5	4	3	2	1
8. I try to see things from the other person's point of view.	5	4	3	2	1
9. I maintain good eye contact when listening.	5	4	3	2	1
10. I get so busy taking notes that I miss some of what is said.	5	4	3	2	1
11. I get distracted easily.	5	4	3	2	1
12. I let my mind wander or I daydream when someone is talking.	5	4	3	2	1

*Adapted from M. M. Brewner, W. C. McMahon, and M. P. Roche. *Job Survival Skills*. New York: Educational Designs, Inc., 1984, p. 64.

ADD THE CIRCLED NUMBERS TO GET YOUR SCORE: _____

45–60   You are a good listener and probably make few mistakes at work. More than likely, people enjoy talking to you and being with you.

31–44   You need to improve your listening skills. This will also improve your job performance.

12–30   You are a poor listener. You have probably lost some friends or made mistakes at work because of your poor listening habits.

Now that you have a score, write out a self-improvement plan of action, if necessary.

TASK 2-4

Recognizing Barriers to Communication*

Objective: To recognize common barriers to effective communication.

Directions: Read each situation statement and match it to the communication barrier it describes.

Communication Barrier Described

a. Criticizing instead of explaining
b. Poor eye contact
c. Ordering instead of asking politely
d. Interrupting
e. Thinking ahead instead of listening

f. Fear of speaking up
g. Misunderstanding
h. Pretending to listen
i. Ignoring what is said
j. Rudely disagreeing

Situation Statements

_____ 1. During break time, several employees were discussing the recent Right to Life protests at the women's clinic. Susan's opinion differed from that of the group. Susan shouted, "You are a bunch of old-fashioned biddies, not liberated." Then she stormed out of the office.

_____ 2. Roger never waits until a person has finished talking. He breaks into conversations with his ideas and never excuses himself.

_____ 3. Rudy was telling Betty about his experience with an angry patient who was upset over a fee for service. Betty looked at Rudy, nodding her head in agreement, but when Rudy asked, "Well what would have said to the patient?" Betty asked, "Rudy, would you repeat what you just said?"

_____ 4. Doctor Parkins told Janna, the medical radiographer, to review the insurance reimbursement on John L. Thomas' X rays. When Janna goes to the files, she finds that Mr. Thomas has had a chest X ray every month for the past year. She wonders if the doctor wants specific information on a particular month or for the entire period.

_____ 5. Supervisor Ellen Brock is giving Marissa directions for opening the office on Saturday. Although she is listening, Marissa is waving to her car-pool companions that she will be out in five minutes.

_____ 6. Robin and Teresa have not been getting along at work. Robin approaches Teresa and says, "I would like to talk with you about our differences." Teresa turns to Helen, another worker, and says, "Where are you going for lunch today?"

_____ 7. Rodney, a limited radiographer, is a new employee and has been asked to perform electrocardiograms (EKG) when he is not busy taking radiographs. Susan has instructed Rodney twice about how to perform an EKG. During an EKG procedure, Rodney has trouble attaching a limb lead and asks Susan for assistance. Susan says, "How many times am I going to have to show you how to do this?"

_____ 8. Joan was telling Becky about her ideas for improving collections on the accounts receivables. Becky keeps thinking, "Wait until she hears my ideas."

_____ 9. Brenda is a new employee in the Springview Medical Clinic. Brenda feels like the clinic supervisor watches every move she makes. This makes Brenda very nervous, but she doesn't know how to tell the supervisor.

_____ 10. Randell, the laboratory assistant, turned from the microscope counter and said, "Jean, get me clean cover slips. I need them right away."

*Adapted from M. M. Brewner, W. C. McMahon, and M. P. Roche. Job Survival Skills. New York: Educational Designs, Inc., 1984, p. 62–63.

TASK 4-1

Procedure: Hand Washing

Terminal Performance Objective: Provided with soap, nail brush, cuticle stick, paper towels, and a waste receptacle, the student will wash his/her hands. All items on the instructor's checklist must be rated satisfactory or not applicable.

Equipment/Supplies

- Soap (Liquid soap dispenser is recommended; however, students need to know the procedure to follow if bar soap is provided.)
- Hot and cold faucets (Students should recognize the different types of faucets available. Hand operated faucets are a source of contamination for clean hands, so a paper towel should be used to turn off the water. Sinks with foot pedal or elbow levers allow the the water to be turned on, off, and regulated without contamination.)
- Nail brush
- Cuticle stick
- Paper towels
- Waste receptacle (preferably foot operated top opener)

Performance Guide

1. Remove all jewelry: rings, bracelets, watches; wedding rings may be left on, but must be scrubbed.

    Key Point: Jewelry that may harbor bacteria should not be worn during work time. If a sterile procedure requiring donning of gloves is to follow hand washing, rings must be left off until after the procedure is completed.

2. Stand in a comfortable position in front of the sink.

    Key Point: Avoid contaminating the uniform by touching the sink or getting it wet. Usually there are many microorganisms around the sink area, because they grow and multiply rapidly in moist surroundings.

3. Adjust water flow and temperature.

    Key Points: If faucets are hand operated, use paper towel to turn them on. Keep water running continuously throughout the hand-washing procedure.

4. Wet hands thoroughly.

    Key Points: Hold hands down toward sink. Water will drain from wrists to fingertips and carry bacteria away.

5. Apply soap.

    Use approximately one teaspoon of a liquid soap from dispenser.

6. Wash hands.
   a. Use circular motion.
   b. Include palms, wrists, back of hands, and fingers of each hand, using strong friction, Figure Ap.4-1A.

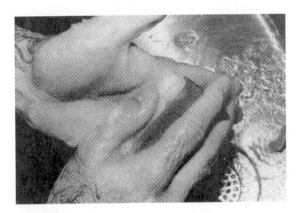

   c. Wash hands approximately two minutes. Prior to donning surgical gloves for assisting with invasive surgical procedures, the surgical scrub procedure must be used. The surgical scrub procedure requires more time in scrubbing than the basic handwashing technique. The length of any handwashing scrub will depend on the frequency of scrubbing, the agent used, and the method. Care must be taken not to abrade the skin during the scrub process.

   Key Points: Use nail brush on nails and all areas of hands and fingers. Use a cuticle stick to remove any material that the brush may not reach under the nails, Figure Ap.4-1B.

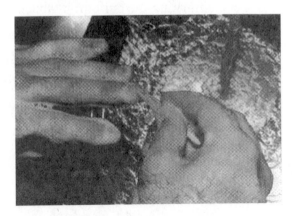

7. Rinse well.

   Key Points: Allow water to run from wrists to fingertips. Avoid touching the inside of the sink.

8. Repeat steps 4–7.

9. Dry hands gently.

10. Turn off water.

    Key Point: If faucets are hand operated, use paper towel to turn off.

    Note: Apply lotion as desired to keep skin soft. Leave the sink and surrounding area neat and dry. A clean, dry environment promotes health.

TASK 4-2

Procedure: Assisting the Falling Patient

Terminal Performance Objective: Provided with a classmate for a patient, assist the falling patient. All items on the instructor's checklist must be marked satisfactory or not applicable.

Equipment/Supplies

■ Classmate as a simulated patient.

Performance Guide

1. Support the patient, holding under the patient's arms. Never try to break the patient's fall because this may increase the possibility of injury.
2. Rest the patient's buttocks against your bent supporting leg.
3. Ease the patient to the floor using the supporting leg.
4. Attend to patient comfort and request assistance.

TASK 4-3

Procedure: Preparing Safety Reports (Accident/Incident)

Terminal Performance Objective: In a simulated safety/accident situation, provided with an accident example and related information, complete a safety and accident report. All items on the instructor's checklist must be rated satisfactory or not applicable.

Equipment/Supplies

- Accident report form
- Simulated accident/safety situation (teacher-prepared scene may be used to role play)

Performance Guide

1. Obtain written log or oral report from persons involved.
2. Complete prescribed accident report forms.
3. Verify written report before it is signed by persons involved.
4. Sign and date forms.
5. Forward original and required number of copies to supervisor.
6. File form copy in departmental file.

TASK 4-4

Procedure: Using a Three-Carrier Lift to Transfer the Patient

Terminal Performance Objective: Provided with a classmate for a patient, three classmate assistants, necessary equipment and supplies, use a three-carrier lift to transfer the patient. All items on the instructor's checklist must be marked satisfactory or not applicable.

Equipment/Supplies

- Classmate as a simulated patient
- Three assistants
- Radiographic table
- Stretcher

Performance Guide

1. Wash hands.
2. Locate and identify the patient.
3. Introduce self and explain procedure.
4. Slide patient to edge of stretcher.
5. Lock stretcher wheels.

6. Position assistants at side of radiographic table:
   - one at patient's head and neck
   - one at patient's buttocks
   - one at legs and ankles
7. Cross patient's arms over chest.
   Persons lifting place their bodies against the area on which patient is lying and place their arms under the patient part they are going to lift.
8. On the count of three, persons lifting roll patient toward their chests.
9. Lifters lift patient and move patient to designated position.
10. Attend to patient comfort.
11. Observe safety precautions.
12. Use good body alignment and mechanics.
13. Repeat procedure in reverse order for transfer back to the stretcher.

TASK 4-5

Procedure: Transferring a Patient Using a Sheet

Terminal Performance Objective: Provided with classmates for a patient and transfer assistants, use a sheet to transfer a patient from a stretcher to the radiographic table. All items on the instructor's checklist must be marked satisfactory or not applicable.

Equipment/Supplies

- Classmate as a simulated patient
- Radiographic table
- Stretcher
- Sheet
- Three to four classmates to serve as transfer assistants.

Performance Guide

1. Wash hands.
2. Explain the procedure to the patient. Talk with the patient. Explain what you will be doing and how he/she can assist.
3. Ask the patient to roll to one side of the stretcher.
4. Fold the sheet in half and place along the patient's backside.
5. Ask the patient to return to his/her back (supine position). The patient will be rolling over the folded sheet.

6. Ask patient to roll to the opposite side (away from the side toward which he/she first rolled).
7. Unfold sheet and smooth out.
8. Ask patient to return to his/her back (supine position).
9. (Need three to four classmates) Position assistant helpers at the following locations:
   - One at patient's head—this person will hold, support, and guide the patient's head during the transfer.
   - One at patient's side.
   - Two across and at side of table onto which patient is to be transferred.
10. All lifters roll transfer sheet up close toward both sides of the patient.
11. In unison, all lifters transfer the patient to the radiographic table.
12. Attend to patient comfort.
13. Observe safety precautions.
14. Use good body alignment and mechanics during the transfer.
15. Repeat procedure in reverse order for transfer back to the stretcher.

TASK 4-6

Procedure: Logrolling the Patient

Terminal Performance Objective: Provided with a classmate for a patient, two assistant helpers, necessary equipment and supplies, logroll a patient onto the radiographic table. All items on the instructor's checklist must be marked satisfactory or not applicable.

Equipment/Supplies

- Classmate as a simulated patient
- Stretcher
- Radiographic table
- Two classmates to serve as assistant helpers

Performance Guide

1. Wash hands.
2. Ask two other assistants to help. Identify the patient and explain what you plan to do.

3. Position assistants. One assistant should be on the same side of the bed as you are. The other assistant should be at the patient's opposite side to keep patient from falling as he/she rolls. If side rails are available on the stretcher, also secure the side rail.

4. Move the patient as a unit toward you. Place a pillow lengthwise between the patient's legs. Fold his/her arms over his/her chest.

5. Turn the patient to his/her side:
   a. Use a turning sheet that has been previously placed under the patient.
      - Reaching over patient, grasp and roll the turning sheet toward the patient.
      - Position one assistant beside the patient to keep shoulders and hips straight. Second assistant should be positioned to keep thighs and lower legs straight.
   b. If a turning sheet is not in position, the first assistant should position hands on far shoulders and hips. Second assistant positions hands on far thigh and lower leg.

6. At a specified signal, the patient is drawn toward both assistants in a single movement, keeping spine, head, and legs in straight position. Additional pillows are placed behind the patient to maintain the position. A small pillow or folded bath blanket may be permitted under the head and neck. Leave pillow between the legs and position small pillows or folded towels to support the arms until ready for radiographic positioning.

7. Check patient for comfort, alignment, and support.

8. Observe all safety precautions.

9. Use good body alignment and mechanics during the transfer.

TASK 4-7

Procedure: Assisting the Patient with Ambulatory Aid: Cane, Walker, and Crutches

Terminal Performance Objective: Provided with a classmate for a patient, assist the patient with an ambulatory aide to move from the waiting area to the radiographic room and on/off the radiographic table. All items on the instructor's checklist must be marked satisfactory or not applicable.

Equipment/Supplies

- Classmate as a simulated patient
- Cane

- Walker
- Crutches
- Radiographic table

Performance Guide

(The simulated situation should pose such obstacles as doors and hallways similar in width to those found in medical facilities.)

1. Wash hands.
2. Locate and identify the patient.
3. Introduce self and briefly explain purpose of transfer.
4. Assess patient's condition.
5. Assist patient to move from waiting area or reception area to radiography room.
6. Assist patient during disrobing, if applicable.
7. Provide support to the patient's weak side as he/she gets onto and off the radiographic table.
8. Provide for patient safety and comfort needs:
   a. Patient with a cane
   b. Patient with a walker
   c. Patient with crutches

TASK 4-8

Procedure: Transporting the Patient in a Wheelchair

Terminal Performance Objective: Provided with a classmate for a patient, a wheelchair, and a beginning and ending destination, transport a patient in a wheelchair. All items on the instructor's checklist must be marked satisfactory or not applicable.

Equipment/Supplies

- Classmate as a simulated patient
- Wheelchair

Performance Guide

1. Locate and identify the patient.

2. Introduce self and explain procedure.
3. Secure patient's clothing/drapes from possible entanglement.
4. Check to be sure tubes, drainage bottles, catheters, etc., are secure.
5. Release hand brake to unlock wheels.
6. Transport the patient along the right side of the hall.
7. Move through door: (if applicable)
   a. Approach closed doorway backwards.
   b. Use one hand to open door and support door open with body as needed.
   c. Pull chair through backwards.
   d. Turn wheelchair to forward after getting through door.
8. Use elevator: (if applicable)
   a. Secure elevator door.
   b. Pull wheelchair onto elevator backward.
   c. Turn wheelchair around and leave elevator pulling wheelchair backward.
9. Make all turns carefully and smoothly to avoid stress or danger to the patient.
10. When destination is reached set hand brake to lock wheels.

TASK 4-9

Procedure: Transferring the Patient Between Radiographic Table and Wheelchair

Terminal Performance Objective: Provided with a classmate for a patient, wheelchair, radiographic table, and a footstool, transfer the patient between the radiographic table and wheelchair without injury to the patient or damage to equipment. All items on the instructor's checklist must be marked satisfactory or not applicable.

Equipment/Supplies

- Classmate as a simulated patient
- Wheelchair
- Radiographic table
- Footstool

Performance Guide

1. Wash hands.
2. Locate and identify the patient.
3. Introduce self and explain procedure.

4. Position wheelchair beside table, facing head of table.
5. Set wheel brakes and raise footrests.
6. Assist patient to sitting position on the examination table with legs dangling and remove sheet.
7. Assist patient to standing position on footstool.
8. Assist patient to step down from footstool.
9. Assist patient to pivot and lower body into wheelchair.
10. Reverse procedure to move patient from wheelchair onto examination table.
11. Cover patient with sheet.
12. Ensure patient is comfortable before leaving.
13. Observe all safety precautions.
14. Use good body alignment and mechanics when transferring patient.

TASK 4-10

Procedure: Preparing Patient for Radiographic Examination

Terminal Performance Objective: In a simulated situation, provided with a classmate as a patient, radiographic request, and examination gown, prepare the patient for a radiographic examination. All items on the instructor's checklist must be rated acceptable or not applicable.

Equipment/Supplies

- Classmate as a simulated patient
- Prepare patient situations on 3" × 5" card so that the simulated patient will be required to present specific patient situations.
- Examination room or privacy screen.
- Radiographic request—request should be for a specific body area that will require the student to request that the patient disrobe. In practice situation, student should be provided with situations that are reality-based—e.g., patient with mastectomy who requires assistance in removing clothing.
- Examination gown.

Performance Guide

1. Review radiographic request.
2. Locate and identify patient.

Key Point: In some medical facilities, the patient may be waiting in the reception room. To avoid miscommunication, use a clear, articulate voice when saying the patient's name. Always ask the patient his/her name. Do not say to a patient, "Are you Mr(s). Smith?" He/she may misunderstand and nod or confirm to the wrong identity.

3. Introduce self and explain procedure.
4. Assess patient's physical ability.

Key Point: Never leave a patient unattended or alone to disrobe if he/she is unstable or seems confused. Never leave young children unattended.

5. Give the patient instructions to disrobe and don examination gown.

Key Point: Be very specific as to what articles of clothing should be removed. Be specific regarding undergarments, jewelry, or any opaque objects.

a. Assist patient in removing clothing.
b. Explain how to put on examination gown.
c. Take care of patient's valuables.

TASK 4-11

Procedure: Taking Temperature by Mercury, Electronic, and Tympanic Thermometers

Terminal Performance Objective: Provided with a classmate for a patient, necessary equipment, and supplies, take and record the patient's oral temperature. Methods of measurement will be a mercury thermometer and an electronic thermometer. All items on the instructor's checklist must be rated satisfactory or not applicable.

Equipment/Supplies

- Classmate as a simulated patient
- Sterilization supplies if thermometers are not disposable
- Oral, glass tube thermometer with elongated tip
- Electronic thermometer with disposable sheath covers
- Blunt tip (short rounded) rectal thermometer (to be used for demonstration only).

Performance Guide

1. Wash hands.
2. Locate and identify the patient.
3. Introduce self and explain procedure to the patient.

4. *Mercury Thermometer*: Pick up thermometer and wipe; if necessary, rinse off antiseptic solution in cool water.

  or

  Electronic Thermometer: Apply sterile protective disposable sheath cover to electronic thermometer.
5. Shake mercury down to 96°F or 36.5°C; or set electronic digital scale.
6. Appropriately insert thermometer.
7. Leave thermometer in place the required amount of time, or until buzzer signals for electronic thermometer.
8. Remove and read scale.
9. Clean thermometer or discard sheath.
10. Replace thermometer in holder.
11. Record patient's temperature.

  Tympanic thermometer

  Complete steps 1–3 in Performance Guide.
1. Place cover on thermometer Figure A-1.
2. Set thermometer to start.
3. Gently place probe into ear canal to seal the area and activate the system Figure A-2.
4. Wait until the temperature appears on the screen.
5. Remove from the ear.

  Complete steps 8–11 in Performance Guide.

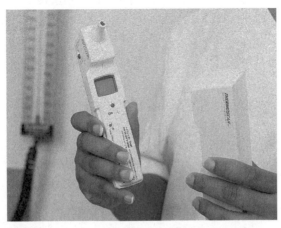

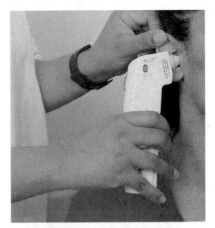

Figure A-1 Attach the disposable speculum or cover to the tympanic thermometer to prevent spread of microorganisms between patients.

Figure A-2 Pull up on the ear to straighten the auditory canal for an accurate reading.

TASK 4-12

Procedure: Counting the Radial Pulse and Respiratory Rate

Terminal Performance Objective: Provided with a classmate for a patient, take and record the patient's radial pulse and respiratory rate. All items on the instructor's checklist must be marked acceptable or not applicable.

Equipment/Supplies

- Classmate as a simulated patient
- Watch with second hand

Performance Guide

1. Wash hands.
2. Locate and identify patient.
3. Place patient in a comfortable position. The palm of the hand should be down and the arm should rest across the patient's chest.
4. Locate the pulse on the thumb side of the wrist with the tips of your first three fingers. Do not use your thumb since it contains a pulse that may be confused with the patient's pulse.
5. When the pulse is felt, exert slight pressure. Use second hand of watch and count for one minute.
6. When the pulse rate has been counted, leave the fingers on the radial pulse and start counting the number of times the chest rises and falls during one minute.
7. Note depth and regularity of respirations.
8. Record the pulse rate, time, rhythm, and the regularity and depth of respirations.

TASK 4-13

Procedure: Taking Blood Pressure

Terminal Performance Objective: Provided with a classmate for a patient and necessary equipment and supplies, take and record the patient's blood pressure. All items on the instructor's checklist must be marked acceptable or not applicable.

Equipment/Supplies

- Classmate as a simulated patient

- Stethoscope
- Blood pressure cuff
- Sphygmomanometer (mercury or aneroid)

Performance Guide

1. Wash hands.
2. Locate and identify the patient.
3. Assemble the equipment needed: sphygmomanometer and stethoscope. (Clean stethoscope earpieces and bell with antiseptic solution.)
4. Place the patient's arm palm-upward, supported on bed or table.
5. Roll sleeve of patient's gown up about five inches above elbow. Be sure it is not tight on the arm.
6. Apply cuff smoothly and evenly one to one-and-one-half inches above the elbow. The center of the rubber bladder should be directly over the brachial artery. The brachial artery is located on the inside of the arm (medial aspect) just inside the elbow. If the cuff is marked with an arrow, place cuff so that the arrow points over the brachial artery.
7. Tuck ends of cuff and hook to secure closure. Be sure cuff is secure but not too tight. Check by slipping two fingers between cuff and patient's arm.
8. Locate the radial artery and palpate it as you:
   a. Close valve attached to hand pump (air bulb) by turning it clockwise.
   b. Quickly inflate cuff until the gauge registers 50 mm Hg.
   c. Continue to inflate cuff in 10-mm-Hg increments until radial pulse cannot be felt. This pressure indicates the palpated systolic pressure. Note the pressure.
   d. Quickly deflate cuff by turning the close valve counterclockwise.
9. Ask the patient to raise the arm and flex fingers.
10. Locate the brachial artery with the fingers.
11. Place earpieces in ears. Place bell of stethoscope directly over the artery.
12. Close valve and reinflate cuff quickly until gauge registers 30 mm above palpated systolic pressure.
13. Listen carefully as you open valve of pump by turning counterclockwise.
14. Let air escape slowly (between 1–3 mm per second) until first heart sound is heard. Note reading on manometer at top of meniscus as the systolic pressure.
15. Continue to release the air pressure slowly until there is an abrupt change of the sound from very loud to a soft muffled sound. The reading at which this change is heard is the diastolic pressure. In some facilities, the last sound heard is taken as the diastolic pressure.

16. Rapidly deflate cuff and remove, expel air from the cuff, and replace apparatus. Clean earpieces and bell of stethoscope with antiseptic solution.

    Note: If repeat procedure is necessary, wait at least one minute.

    a. As patient to raise arm and flex fingers.

    b. Repeat procedure.

17. Remember to wash your hands, report completion of task, and document date, time, systolic and diastolic readings as an improper fraction, patient's reaction, and site of reading if other than the brachial artery.

TASK 7-1

Procedure: Cleaning Radiographic Facilities and Equipment

Terminal Performance Objective: Given a radiographic room, clean the facilities and equipment. Area must be clean and free of dust.

Equipment/Supplies

- Radiographic equipment (table, tube stand console)
- Cleaning solutions
- Cleaning cloths
- Gloves (if needed to protect hands)

Performance Guide

1. Place dampened or wet items, such as dressings and bandages, in waterproof bags and close bags tightly before discarding.
2. Dust mechanical parts of the X-ray machine with a clean, damp (not wet) cloth.
3. Clean table with a disinfectant beginning with the least dirty to the most dirty area.
4. Clean metal parts with benzine or a solution specified by the hospital procedure manual.
5. Polish metal parts.
6. Clean overhead parts (X-ray tube and other parts that conduct electricity) with alcohol or a clean, dry cloth.

    CAUTION: Never use water to clean electrical parts.

    Note: Clean cones, compression devices, and other accessories daily.

7. Dissolve adhesive-tape residue from cassettes with benzine, then wash with alcohol or warm soapy water.
8. Put fresh linen on table and pillow.

   Note: Make sure that rags and mops are disinfected and dried before reuse.

TASK 7-2

Procedure: Operating Radiographic Tables and Consoles

Terminal Performance Objective: Provided with a classmate for a patient and necessary equipment and supplies, perform the functions listed in the performance guide.

Equipment/Supplies

- Buckey tray
- Cassettes
- Student (to act as patient)
- Tissue caliper

Performance Guide

Each student will
1. Properly place various sizes of cassettes in the buckey tray.
2. Properly align the CR with the table top and with the film (cassette) in the bucky tray.
3. Raise and lower the table with a patient (another student) on the table.
4. Use a caliper to measure various parts of another student. Use supine and standing positions.

TASK 9-1

Procedure: Testing Safelight Performance

Terminal Performance Objective: Given a cassette, radiographic film, radiographic equipment, and a film processor, determine whether the safelight is fogging the film. All items on the instructor's checklist must be rated satisfactory or not applicable.

Equipment/Supplies

- Cassette
- Radiographic film (exposed)
- Radiographic equipment (energized)
- Film processor
- Safelight illuminator

Performance Guide

1. Select two cassettes loaded with film.
2. Expose each to a very minimal X-ray exposure (about 10.0 mAs, 60 kv, 40" SID).

   Note: Both cassettes must receive exactly the same exposure.
3. Remove the film from one cassette under conditions that normally exist in the darkroom and process the film.
4. Turn off safelight(s) and remove the film from the remaining cassette.

   Note: This step must be accomplished in total darkness.
5. Process the film.
6. Check the film for differences in density by placing side by side on the same viewbox.

TASK 9-2

Procedure: Maintaining Master Card File or Computer System

Terminal Performance Objective: Provided with a master card file system or a computer terminal, a listing of examinations performed, and necessary patient data, enter the information on the card file or computer file. Each entry must include the patient's name, identification number, age, birth date, examination name, date, X-ray file number, and the physician's and operator's names. All items on the instructor's checklist must be marked satisfactory or not applicable.

Equipment/Supplies

- Pen/pencil
- Master cards or computer system information
- Master card files or computer file

- Patient's chart
- Daily examination record

Performance Guide

1. Obtain patient's updated medical file.
2. Locate patient's master card (file on computer).
   Note: If no master card or computer file exists, the operator must create one. (See step 3 for required information.)
3. Remove master card and record update information or record updated information in computer file:
   a. patient's name and age/birth date
   b. patient's identification number
   c. examination name and date
   d. X-ray file number
   e. physician's name
   f. operator's name
4. Verify that update information is correct.
5. Place master card in correct location according to filing system used or store computer information properly.

TASK 9-3

Procedure: Indexing and Filing Radiographs

Terminal Performance Objective: Given radiographs and film folders, index and file them according to the established filing system. All items must be filed in the patient's folder according to the established filing system. All items on the instructor's checklist must be marked satisfactory or not applicable.

Equipment/Supplies

- Radiographic requests
- Radiographs
- Filing/index system
- Storage receptacle
- Interpretation records

Performance Guide

1. Determine the system of filing:
   a. numerical
   b. alphabetical
   c. disease code index
   d. color code
2. Check for previous radiographs or examinations.
3. Index the folder(s) by writing identifying information on the film folders.
   a. patient name
   b. examination
   c. patient number
   d. date
   e. physician
4. Place radiograph(s) and folder(s) in the diagnostic reading area.
5. After diagnostic interpretation, place radiographs in corresponding film folder(s).
6. File the folder(s).

TASK 9-4

Procedure: Processing Loans of Radiographs

Terminal Performance Objective: Given a request for a loan of radiographs, process the radiographs for loan. All information must be recorded on the mailing folder and the patient's permanent folder without error. All items on the instructor's checklist must be marked satisfactory or not applicable.

Equipment/Supplies

- Loan request
- Radiographs
- Master card file system
- Requested radiographs

Performance Guide

1. Retrieve film to be loaned; determine return due date.
2. Place duplicates of the radiographs in a loan folder.

3. Write patient's name, radiographic number, and physician's name on loan folder.
4. Address folder; include return address.
5. Record the following: date, to whom films were loaned (complete address), and number and size of films sent. Also note the return due date on patient's permanent folder and in the patient's medical file, where applicable.

TASK 9-5

Procedure: Loading and Unloading a Cassette

Terminal Performance Objective: Provided with a cassette, film, and a darkroom environment, load and unload the cassette. The film must not be fogged nor contain artifacts. The intensifying screen must be free of damage. All items on the instructor's checklist must be marked satisfactory or not applicable.

Equipment/Supplies

- Cassette (authors suggest providing student practice with the following: hinge cassette and two pressure bar cassettes)
- X-ray film
- Darkroom environment

Performance Guide

1. Place cassette, with exposed film on work area.
2. Close darkroom door, turn off white lights.
3. Turn on safelight.
4. Open film holder. (See note under equipment and supplies regarding practice with a variety of film holders.)
5. Tip front of cassette.
   Note: This tipping allows the film to fall free of the cassette borders.
6. Grasp film gently at an edge or corner.
7. Lift film out of film holder.
8. Grasp film on corner opposite of side of film being lifted. (This avoids a kink mark in the film.)
9. Insert film into printer. (The next step, processing the film, should be used only if student is ready for this step.)

Reloading a cassette:

10. Open film bin or storage container.
11. Grasp unexposed film with thumb and forefinger.
12. Lift out of film box/bin.
13. Grasp bottom edge with thumb and forefinger of other hand.
14. Load cassette using both hands.
15. Close or secure cassette.
16. Place loaded film holder with other unexposed cassettes.
17. Check to determine if film bin is closed or film safely covered.
18. Turn on white lights.
19. Open door and exit.

TASK 9-6

Procedure: Cleaning Intensifying Screens

Terminal Performance Objective: Given a cassette, screen cleaner, and a cleaning cloth, clean the intensifying screen. Screen must not be nicked, scratched, or chipped while being cleaned, and must be free of smudges and foreign particles. All items on the instructor's checklist must be marked satisfactory or not applicable.

Equipment/Supplies

- Cassette
- Screen cleaner (use commercial brand recommended by screen manufacturer)
- Soft, lint-free cloth

Performance Guide

1. Turn off white lights and turn on safelight.
2. Unload cassette in darkroom (follow directions for handling film). Put unexposed film in film bin or storage container. Secure film bin from light exposure.
3. Turn white lights on.
4. Check screens for dust or foreign materials.
5. Wipe screens with screen cleaner.
   a. Pour cleaner onto soft cloth. *Do not pour solution on screens.*
   b. Rub gently in circular direction. Overlap strokes.
   c. Care must be taken not to nick, scratch, or chip the screens.
6. Dry screen with lint-free cloth.

7. Stand the half-opened cassette on its side for about one-half hour in a dust-free room for further drying. If the cassette screen has been numbered for future film identification matching, these numbers may require remarking after cleaning.* Check to determine that the inside cassette number matches the number on the outside of the cassette.
8. Reload cassette with unexposed film.
9. Record cassette number, date cleaned, and any significant findings.
10. If screen appears damaged, report to appropriate supervisor.

TASK 9-7

Procedure: Testing Cassette for Screen-Film Contact (See Figure 9-12.)

Terminal Performance Objective: Given a cassette, radiographic film, a wire mesh or screen, radiographic equipment and processor, perform a screen-film contact test. Determine whether the cassette has proper screen-film contact. All items on the instructor's checklist must be marked satisfactory or not applicable.

Equipment/Supplies

- Cassette(s)
- Wire mesh or screen (sized to cover entire front of the cassette being tested)
- Radiographic equipment (energized)
- Radiographic processor
- Radiographic film

Performance Guide

1. Assemble supplies and cassettes in radiographic room.
2. Place wire mesh or screen over cassette. Cassette should be positioned under X-ray beam.
3. Set exposure factors (usually 50 kvp, $\frac{1}{20}$ second, 50 mA, 40 in SID).
4. Make exposure.
5. Process film.

Note: If unwanted shadows or artifacts appear on the finished radiograph, having a number on the screen and on the outside of the cassette will help to quickly locate the cassette in question.

6. Check radiograph for areas of blurring.*
7. Record findings. A log should be maintained that contains the number of the cassette tested, the date, and the results. Any areas of blurring should be reported to supervisor.
8. Straighten the work area.

TASK 9-8

Procedure: Processing Film by Manual Method (See Figure 9-17)

Terminal Performance Objective: Provided with manual processing tanks, thermometer, stir stick, timer, processing hanger, a darkroom environment, and a film holder containing exposed film, process the film in manual processing tanks. The film must be free of artifacts and must not be fogged. All items on the instructor's checklist must be marked satisfactory or not applicable.

Equipment/Supplies

- Cassette containing exposed film
- Manual processing tanks
- Thermometer
- Stir sticks (one for developer and one for fixer)
- Timer
- Darkroom environment

Performance Guide

1. Assemble all necessary supplies.
2. Close darkroom door and secure.
3. Stir developer solution.
   - Check water temperature using thermometer.
   - Determine development and fixation time.
   - Stir solutions.
   - Determine if chemical level and activity is sufficient for processing.

Note: It is easier to stand five to six feet back from the viewing illuminator. At this distance, blurred areas will stand out as areas of darker density. If a blurred area appears, it indicates that the screen is warped. The cassette must be repaired or discarded. Today, most manufacturers recommend that the cassette be discarded.

4. Mix stop bath solution, if available. (Always use clean stir stick.)
5. Mix fixer solution.
6. Read chemical thermometer.*
7. Determine development time.*
8. Determine fixation time.*
9. Set processing timer, but do not start.
10. Turn off white lights and turn on safelight.
11. Unload cassette.
12. Load wire hanger.
13. Immerse film in developer solution and start the timer.
14. Agitate film gently to dislodge air bubbles.
15. Remove film from developer when timer goes off. (Do not drain in tank.)
16. Rinse film in wash bath for thirty seconds. Allow excess water to drain off.
17. Immerse film in fixer solution and start the timer.
18. Agitate film gently to dislodge air bubbles.
19. Remove film from solution when timer goes off.
20. Rinse film in final wash for twenty to thirty minutes, depending upon the rate of water exchange (recommended rate of water exchange is eight times per hour).
21. Suspend hanger in dryer or drip rack.
22. Clip the corners of the dry radiograph. This prevents snagging on other films.
23. Straighten work area. Reload film holder in darkroom environment.

TASK 9-9

Procedure: Processing Film by Automatic Method

Terminal Performance Objective: Provided with an automatic processor, a darkroom environment, and a cassette containing exposed film, process the film using the automatic processor. The film must be free of artifacts and must not be fogged. All items on the instructor's checklist must be marked satisfactory or not applicable.

Note: Determine by using manufacturer's suggested time/temperature guidelines. (See Figure 9-18.)

Equipment/Supplies

- Exposed radiograph in cassette
- Safelight illumination
- Automatic processor
- Darkroom environment

Performance Guide

1. Enter darkroom, turn off white light.
2. Check for white-light leaks.
3. Turn on safelight illuminator.
4. Open cassette.
5. Remove film and place on feed tray according to manufacturer's recommendations.
   CAUTION: Do not touch face of film. Grasp film by edges.
6. Push film forward until it is caught by rollers.
   Note: Bell will ring or a dimly lit flasher light will flash to indicate that the film is completely in the processor and replenishment has stopped.
7. Reload cassette.
8. Secure door on film bin and turn on white lights.
9. Open door and exit.
10. Retrieve processed film when it emerges from processor.